THE SICK OF BEING SICK BOOK

Also by Jovial Bob Stine

How To Be Funny
The Absurdly Silly Encyclopedia & Fly Swatter
The Pigs' Book of World Records

Also by Jane Stine

Investigating: Gathering Information

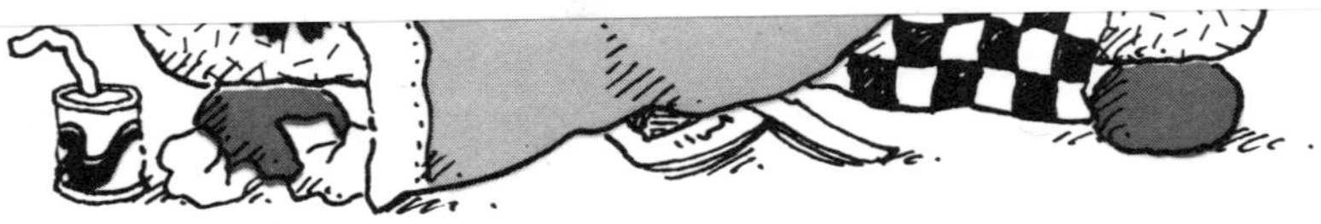

E. P. DUTTON • NEW YORK

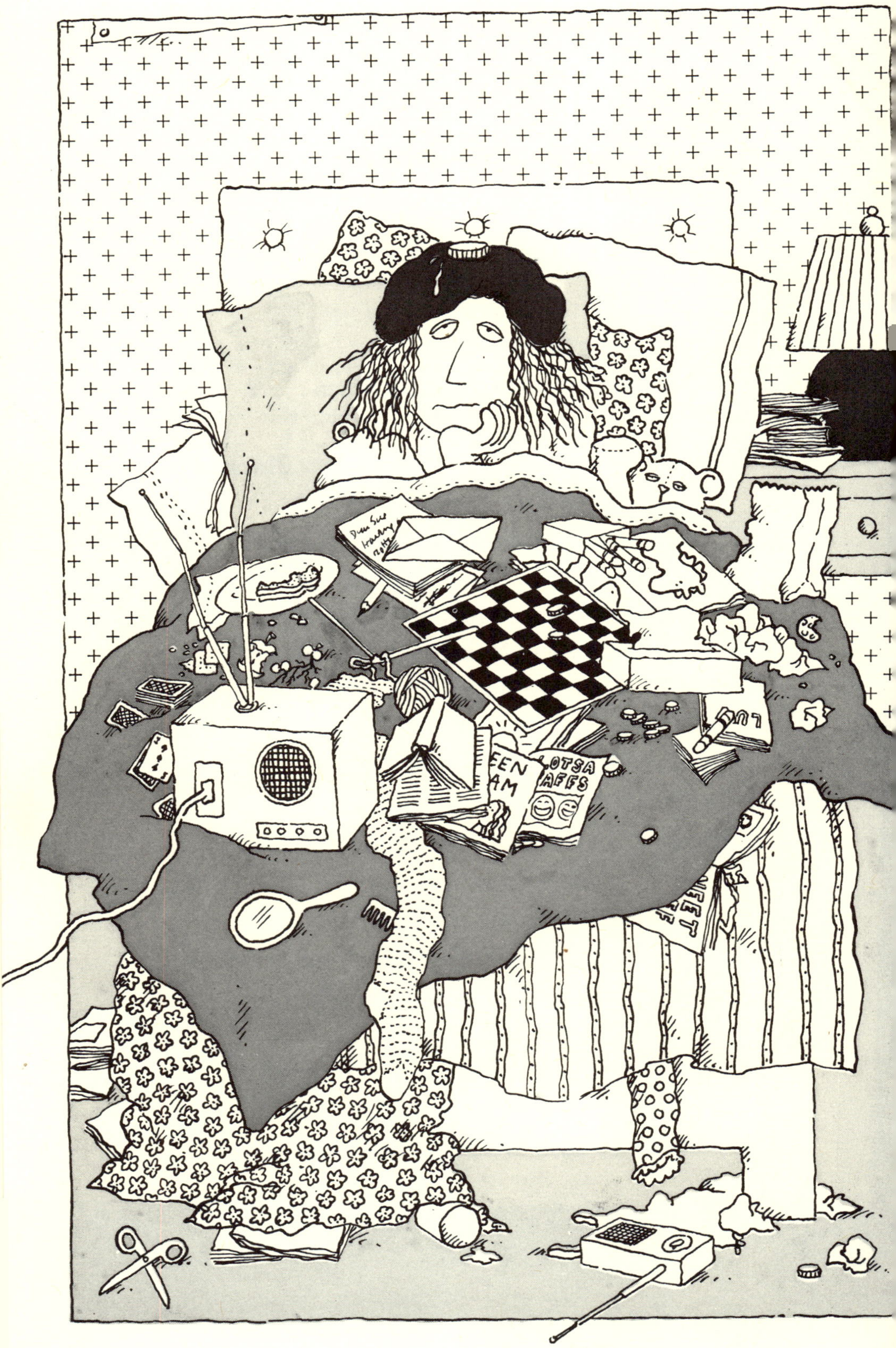

Introduction

Gee, you look terrible!

And you feel as bad as you look, right?

Well, look at the bright side—you only get sick a couple of times a year, so you might as well make the most of it!

No, we don't mean you should spend your time doing the kind of boring projects other books suggest. We know that when you're sick, you're just not interested in building a replica of your uncle out of toothpicks or learning the chords to 300 folk songs you can hum with a runny nose. When you're sick, you want to concentrate on only one thing—how crummy you feel!

And that's what *The Sick of Being Sick Book* is all about—*being sick!* And being sick of being sick. And being sick of being sick of being sick!

So put away the toothpicks, stow the macaroni beads, and get rid of the red construction paper. Being sick is no fun. We know that. But with *The Sick of Being Sick Book* around, at least it can be pretty funny!

You Know You're Getting Sick When . . .

You know you're getting sick when . . .
Someone offers you a candy bar and you hear yourself say, "No thanks. I'm still full from the hard-boiled egg I couldn't finish at lunch!"

You know you're getting sick when . . .
You'd rather rub an ice cube on your forehead than put it down a friend's back!

You know you're getting sick when . . .
Your hair hurts!

You know you're getting sick when . . .
You keep falling asleep in the middle of a football game—and you're the quarterback!

You know you're getting sick when . . .
You ask your mother to turn down the radio—and she tells you it isn't on!

You know you're getting sick when . . .
Your clothes feel heavy!

You know you're getting sick when . . .
You find yourself putting on two sweaters and an overcoat to go to the July 4th picnic!

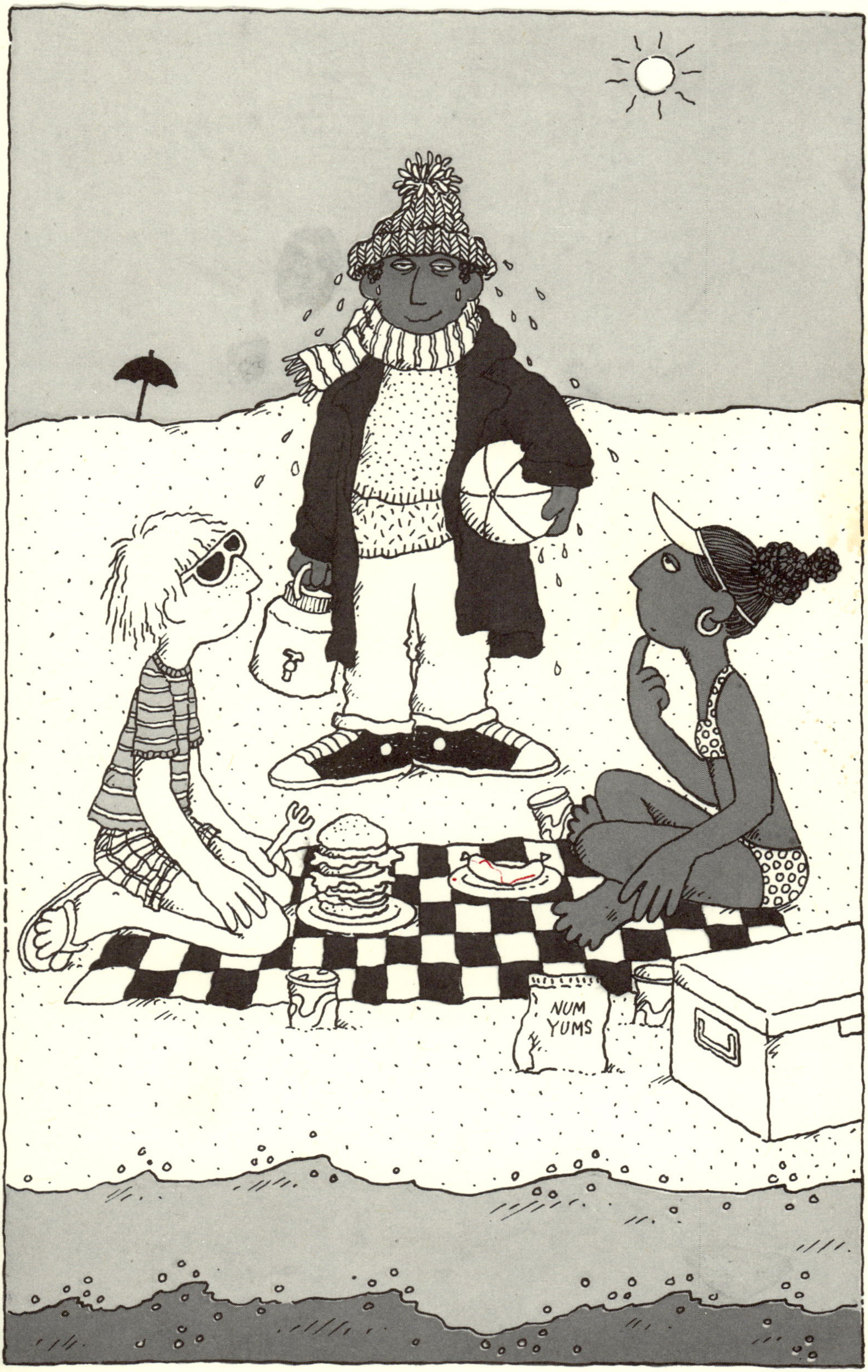
NUM
YUMS

You know you're getting sick when . . .
You wake up in the middle of the night and can't figure out how to get out of bed!

You know you're getting sick when . . .
You compliment a friend on his polka-dot shirt—and he tells you his shirt is plain white!

You know you're getting sick when . . .
You have a wild craving for tea and toast!

A Get Well Card for You

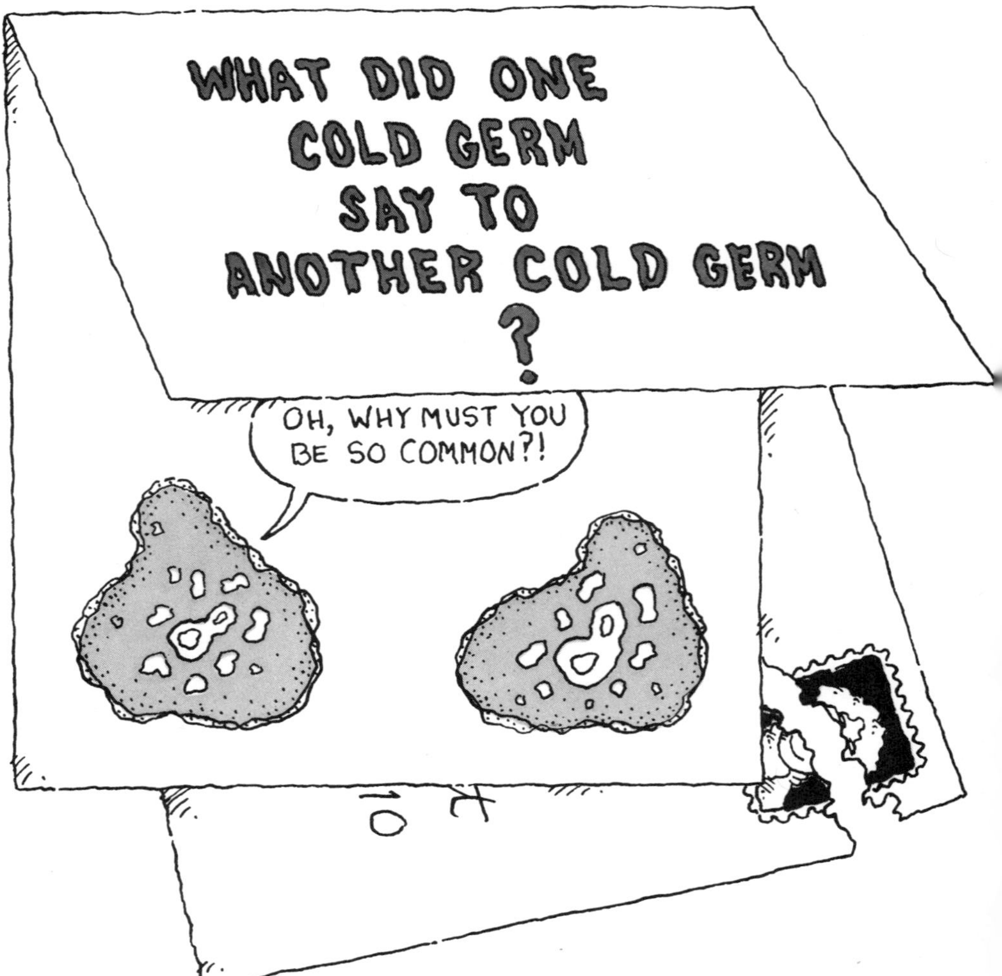
WHAT DID ONE COLD GERM SAY TO ANOTHER COLD GERM ?
OH, WHY MUST YOU BE SO COMMON?!
TO

How To Get the Most Sympathy From Your Illness

You're sick, and naturally your family is trying hard to cheer you up.

"Keep your chin up—you'll be fine again in no time!"

"Stop worrying—you don't look so sick to me!"

This is *not* what you want to hear. You want *sympathy!*

How can you get the most sympathy from your illness? This chapter will help you turn those cries of "You look better already" into groans of "Oh, you poor thing!"

YOU'RE AS SICK AS YOUR CLOTHING

You have to *look* sick to get the kind of heartfelt sympathy you want and need. And you'll never look sick as long as you stay in your regular school clothes.

An Important Rule: Get into pajamas as soon as possible. When you feel that first tickle in your throat, that first ache in your back—reach for the pajamas.

Be careful which pair of pajamas you select. Stay away from bright, cheerful colors. You want to get comments on your cough—not on your wardrobe!

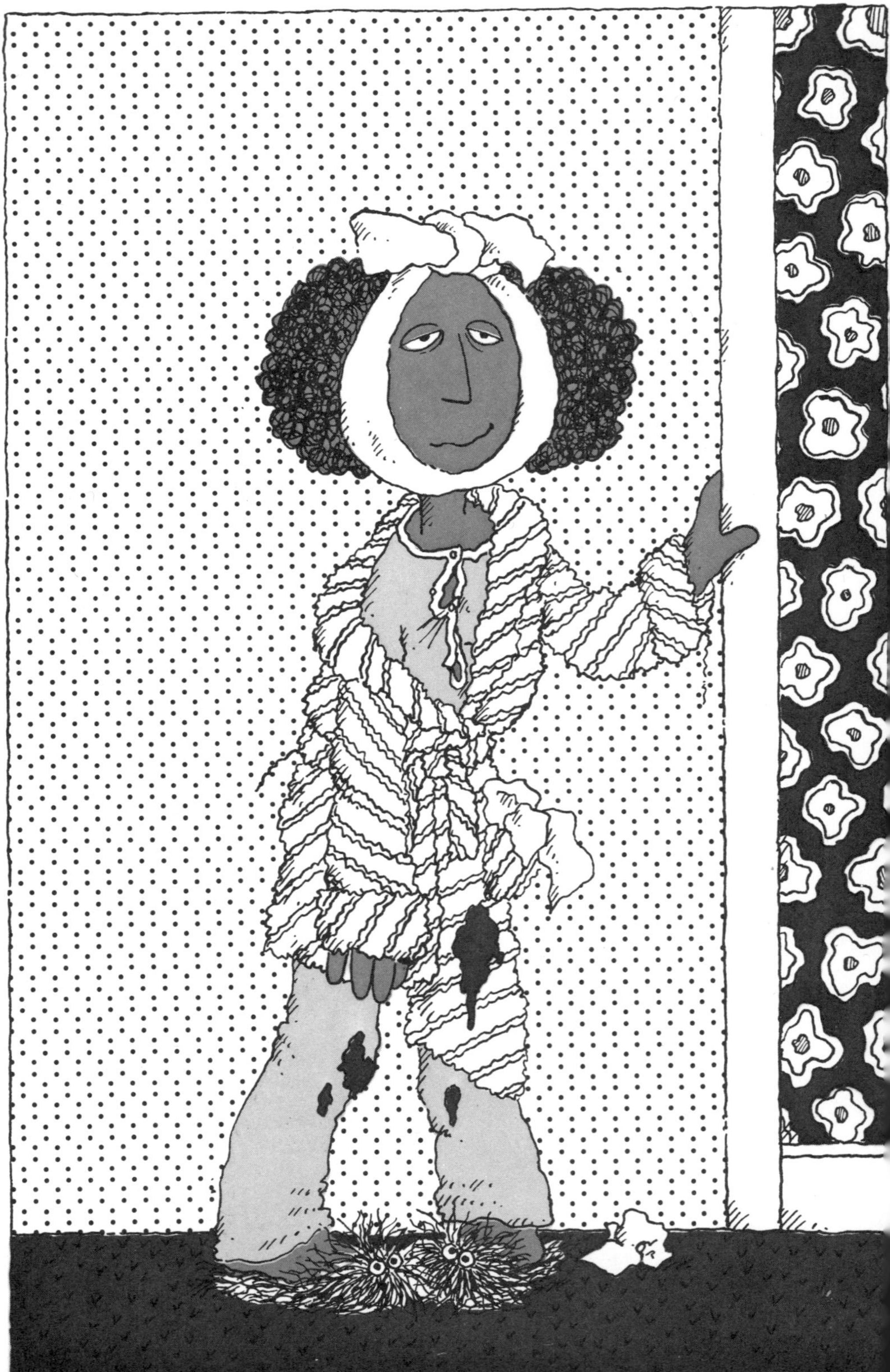

Stick with the drabbest, grayest pair of pj's you can find. A few mysterious stains down the front will help. If you are trying to get sympathy for an upset stomach, wear light green pajamas to highlight the green tones in your skin. If you have the measles or chicken pox, wear pajamas with red polka dots.

Do your best to look as uncomfortable as possible in your pajamas. If necessary, wear the top on bottom and the bottom on top.

DON'T HAVE WORDS TO DESCRIBE IT!

It's a weekday morning and you don't feel too well. You are eager to get a little sympathy from your mother—and the day off from school as well! Perhaps you are a little too eager. Read the following dialogue. See if you can spot your error.

Mother: Good morning. How are you this morning?
You: Not too well. I seem to be suffering from an acute inflammation of the nasopharynx, complicated by severe congestion of the upper respiratory tract and bilateral occlusion of the eustachian tubes.
Mother: That's nice, dear. Have a good day in school.

What did you do wrong?

Answer: You were trying too hard. How sick could you be if you could remember words like *occlusion* and *nasopharynx* before breakfast?

Practice your muttering. Practice slurring your words, letting the sounds roll down your chin and into your shirt. If you're really desperate, move your lips without making any sounds. The person who originally said that silence is golden was probably trying to get a day off from school!

THE SYMPATHY EQUATION

It's important to memorize this simple equation: Bravery = Sympathy. What's the easiest way to show that you are struggling to be brave despite your illness? Never answer a question. If possible, always answer a question with another question. For example:

Mother: How are you feeling, dear?
You: Why worry yourself, Mom?
Mother: Are you sneezing?
You: Isn't it nice and warm in here?
Mother: You're warm? Do you have a fever?
You: Do polar bears really like to sleep on ice?
Mother: Oh, you poor, poor thing!

THINGS TO SAY THAT WILL ALWAYS WIN YOU SYMPATHY

- Could you please lift up that tissue for me?
- I don't really mind missing the school play which I rehearsed six weeks for.
- I'm hungry. Do you think you could get me a cup of tea and half a piece of toast?
- Could we turn off the TV? I think I'd better rest my eyes.

SOME OTHER TIPS

- Walking into walls is out. This will only get you laughs, not sympathy. The same goes for wearing a Band-Aid over your mouth or wearing a cast over your head!
- If at all possible, try to avoid the following: white powder on your face to make you look paler, fake splints and casts, plastic scabs and artificial wounds, ripped clothing,

and bent coat hangers inside your shirt to make you look hunched over. Remember, you're trying for a little sympathy—not an Academy Award!

- Forget about crying. Crying only annoys people. Instead, act as if you would *like* to cry but are bravely holding back the tears. A simple sniffle, if done with the proper gusto, can be tremendously effective.
- Make sure that people see you attempting to look your best despite how awful you feel. Sit up in bed every ten minutes or so and let people see you struggling to brush your hair.
- Hold on to the wall as you walk, pausing every fourth step to catch your breath. If this doesn't get you sympathy, nothing will. Give up—and go outside and play!

Make Your Own Thermometer!

Here's how to save money by making your own thermometer. It's easy and fun—and a good activity for when you're forced to stay in bed!

You will need:

16 quarts of fine-grained sand
1 gas jet
1 glassblower's mask and gloves
1 50-ton glazier's oven with a 400°F. capacity
2 pounds of untreated mercury
1 gallon of sealant
1 lithographic printing press
12 quarts of red ink
12 quarts of black ink
1 quart of orange juice

Heat the sand and treat it to form glass. Hold the glass over the gas jet and shape it to form a thermometer. Be sure to wear your mask and gloves. Bake the glass in the oven at 350°F. until it is done. Insert the proper amount of mercury and seal tightly. Run the thermometer through the printing press and print the numbers and notches on the side. Drink the orange juice. You must be thirsty.

Total cost: $152,000

Use it in good health!

Test Yourself!

What's Your PQ (Patient Quotient)?

What kind of patient are you? The strong, silent, grin-and-bear-it type or the fear-the-worst, good-bye-cruel-world type? This painless quiz will help you find out!

Just take out a sheet of paper, number from 1 to 10—then write down the letter of the best answer for each question. After you've answered all the questions, check your results in the How To Score Yourself section that follows the test.

Finding your PQ is our Rx for a lot of laughs!

1. **Your mother asks, "Can I bring you anything to eat or drink?" You say:**
A. "No. Just seeing the faces of those I love is enough to sustain me in my hour of need."
B. "No, don't fuss. But if you happen to feel like whipping up some mock turtle soup, beef Wellington, and crepes suzette, I might have a bite!"
C. "No, I'm feeding the entire population of Pittsburgh with what you've brought me already!"

2. **When the doctor asks you to stick out your tongue, you say:**
A. "Okay, I can stick it out—but I'm not sure I have the strength to pull it back in!"
B. "My tongue's okay, Doc. It's supposed to be striped, isn't it?"
C. "Aaaaah."

3. **When your temperature reaches 102, you:**
A. insist you really are sick and decide to play only five innings of baseball instead of nine!
B. call your friends and tell them you got over a hundred. So *what* if they think you're talking about the math test!
C. figure out to whom you're going to leave your comic-book collection.

4. **The doctor says, "You're the eighth case of this I've seen this week." Your first thought is:**
A. Shucks, now I won't have a disease named after me!
B. Yes, I try to keep up with what's in style!
C. I didn't know horses *get* human diseases!

5. **When a rash breaks out on your body, you:**
A. immediately change pajamas since stripes and dots don't go together.
B. say, "Well, at least I don't look so pale anymore!"
C. grab a crayon and play Connect the Dots!

6. **When your little brother comes down with what you've got, you:**
A. tell him, "Don't say I never gave you anything!"
B. challenge him to an Olympic Coughing Competition!
C. agree to sell him your get well cards—at a reasonable price!

7. **When the doctor tells you to drink plenty of liquids, you say:**
A. "Oh, really? I wanted to try drinking solids for a change!"
B. "If I drink any more liquid, I'll need a lifeguard to get into bed!"
C. "Okay. Is a hot fudge sundae a liquid?"

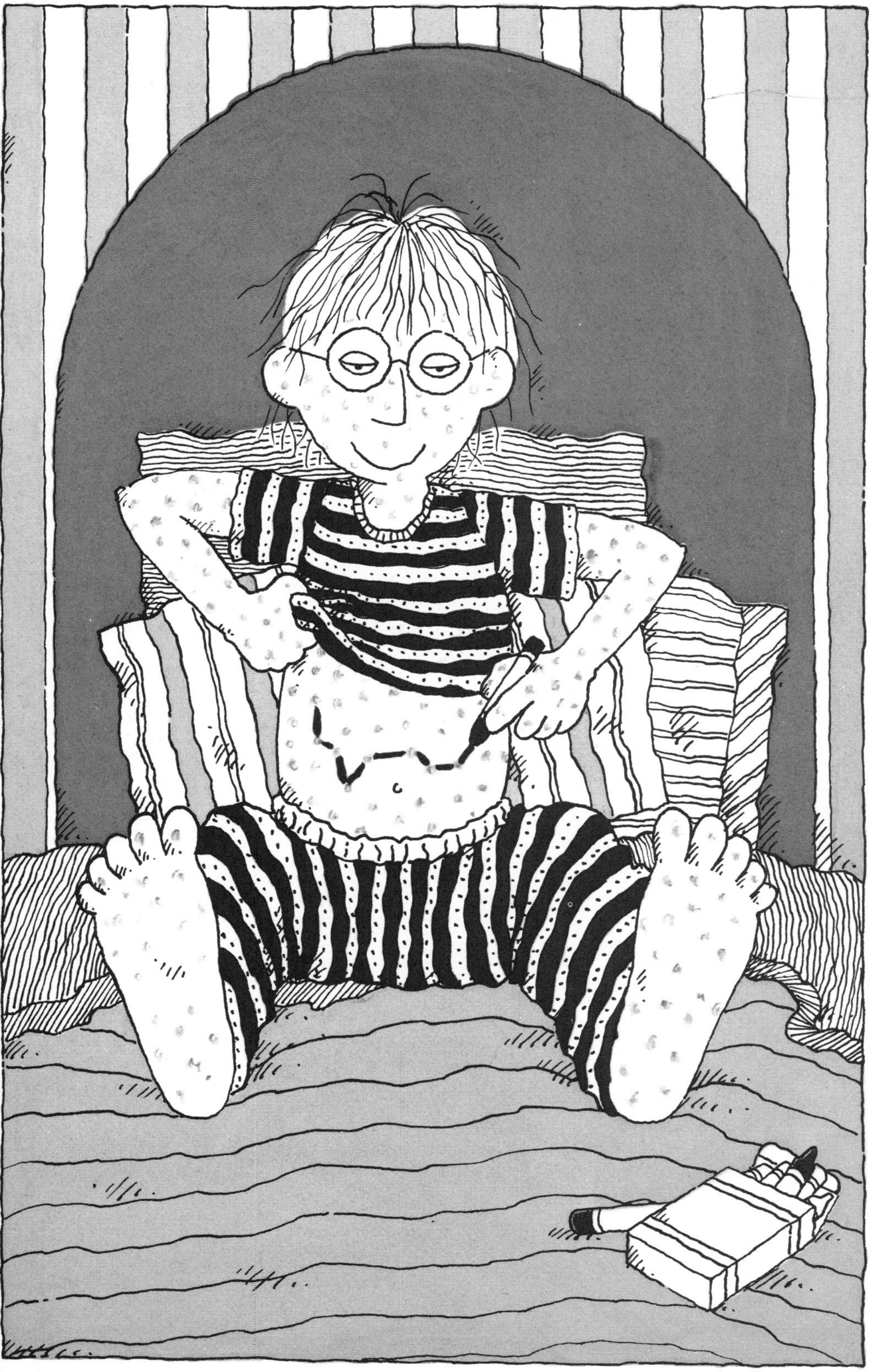

8. **Someone asks, "How are you feeling today?" You say:**
A. "Aside from the throbbing pain, continual agony, and constant discomfort, I feel great!"
B. "Same as yesterday—with my hands!"
C. "About as good as a centipede with swollen ankles!"

9. **The doctor says, "I'm afraid I'm going to have to give you a shot." You say:**
A. "I don't know what *you're* afraid of—*I'm* the one that's getting the shot!"
B. "I'm sorry. I'm opposed to all forms of violence!"
C. "Why don't you give it to my sister instead? She didn't get anything for Christmas!"

10. **When the doctor says you're well enough to go back to school, you:**
A. clutch your heart and say, "Thank you for letting me spend my few remaining days among my friends!"
B. start composing your absence excuse, using such phrases as "miracle cure," "close shave," and "should avoid stress and strain and math homework"!
C. have a relapse!

HOW TO SCORE YOURSELF

Give yourself 5 points for every time you chose *A*. Give yourself 10 points for every time you chose *B*. Give yourself 15 points for every time you had a hard time choosing between *A* and *B*, and chose *C* instead. Give yourself 20 points for every time you chose *C* when you actually meant to choose *A*. Give yourself 10 points for every question you skipped over, meant to go back to, but didn't. Give yourself 15 points if you realized right away that this test is ridiculous. Add up your points and check the rating chart on page 15.

Rating Chart

90–100 points Congratulations! You are an excellent patient. You are courageous, quiet, and cooperative. You'd be absolutely perfect if you didn't have just one flaw—you've got to learn to stop swallowing the thermometer!

75–89 points You're not a bad patient, but you've got a few things to learn. For one thing, your *head* goes on the pillow—not your feet. The next time the doctor asks you to stick out your tongue, swallow your sandwich first!

50–74 points You didn't score too highly, but don't be discouraged. With the proper training and a lot of hard work, you could possibly be a patient for the rest of your life. Good luck!

0–49 points You didn't really score *this* poorly, did you? Why don't you go back and change a few answers so that your score will be higher? You're not such a bad patient, actually. And you'll do a lot better on this test once you learn to lie *in* the bed—not under it!

Don't Just Lie There—
Do Something (#1)

Write Now Word Race
A Pencil Game To Pass the Time

Are you getting a little too good at hitting the wastepaper basket with your wadded-up tissues? Then maybe you're ready for a game that's a little more challenging.

You can play this word game alone or with any number of friends. All you do is select a long word and write it in the center of a piece of paper. Then take three minutes to see how many words you can build from the word you started with. Your new words can go up, down, or across—but they must all relate to your starting word.

Take a look at the following page for an example using the word *thermometer:*

If you're playing with others, the winner is the one who has built the most words after three minutes. If you're playing by yourself, keep a record of the number of words you build, and try to beat your own record.

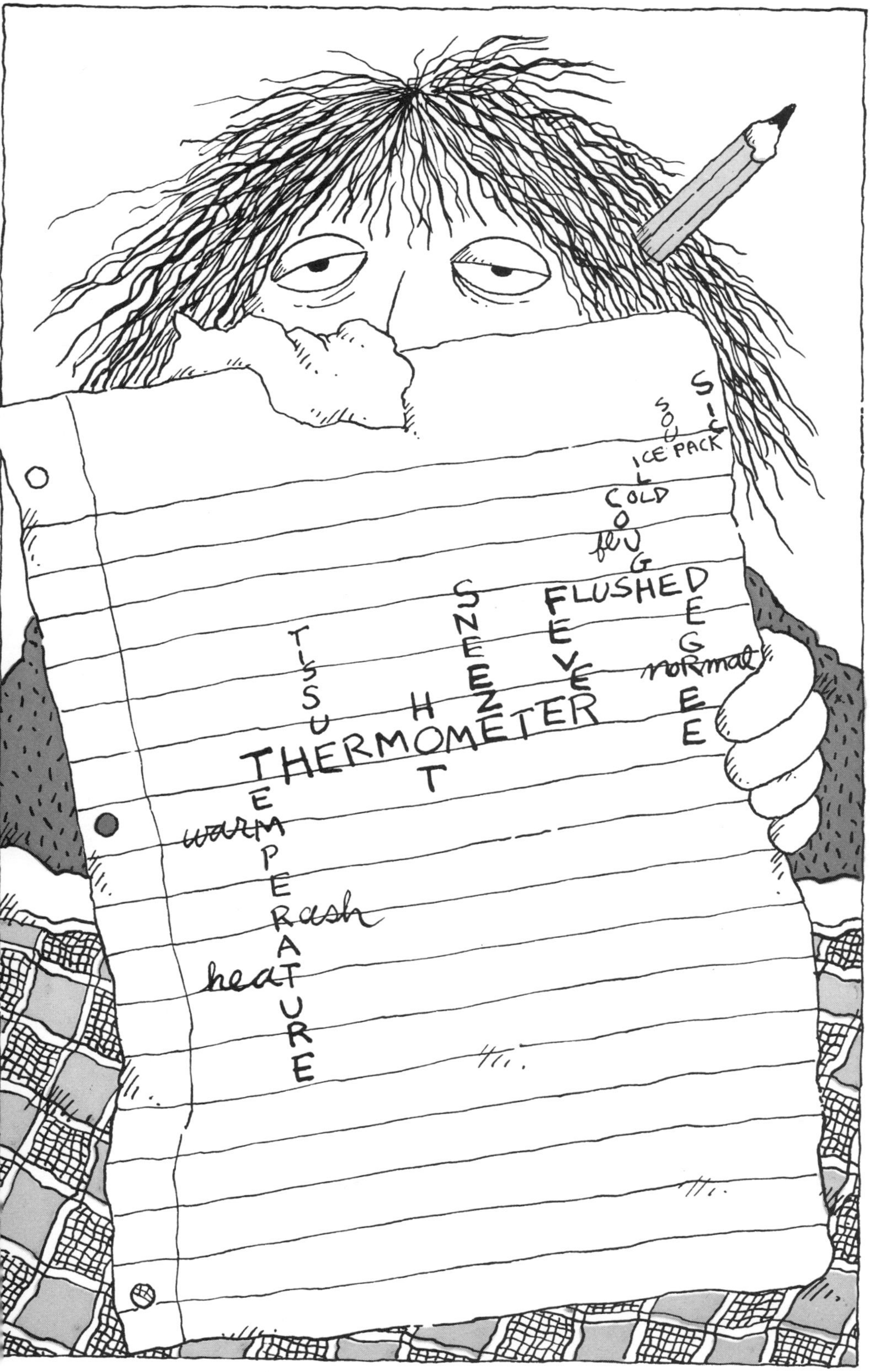
THERMOMETER
TEMPERATURE
TISSUE
HOT
SNEEZE
FEVER
FLUSHED
DEGREE
normal
COUGH
flu
COLD
ICE PACK
SOUP
SICK
warm
rash
heat

A Get Well Card From Your Dog

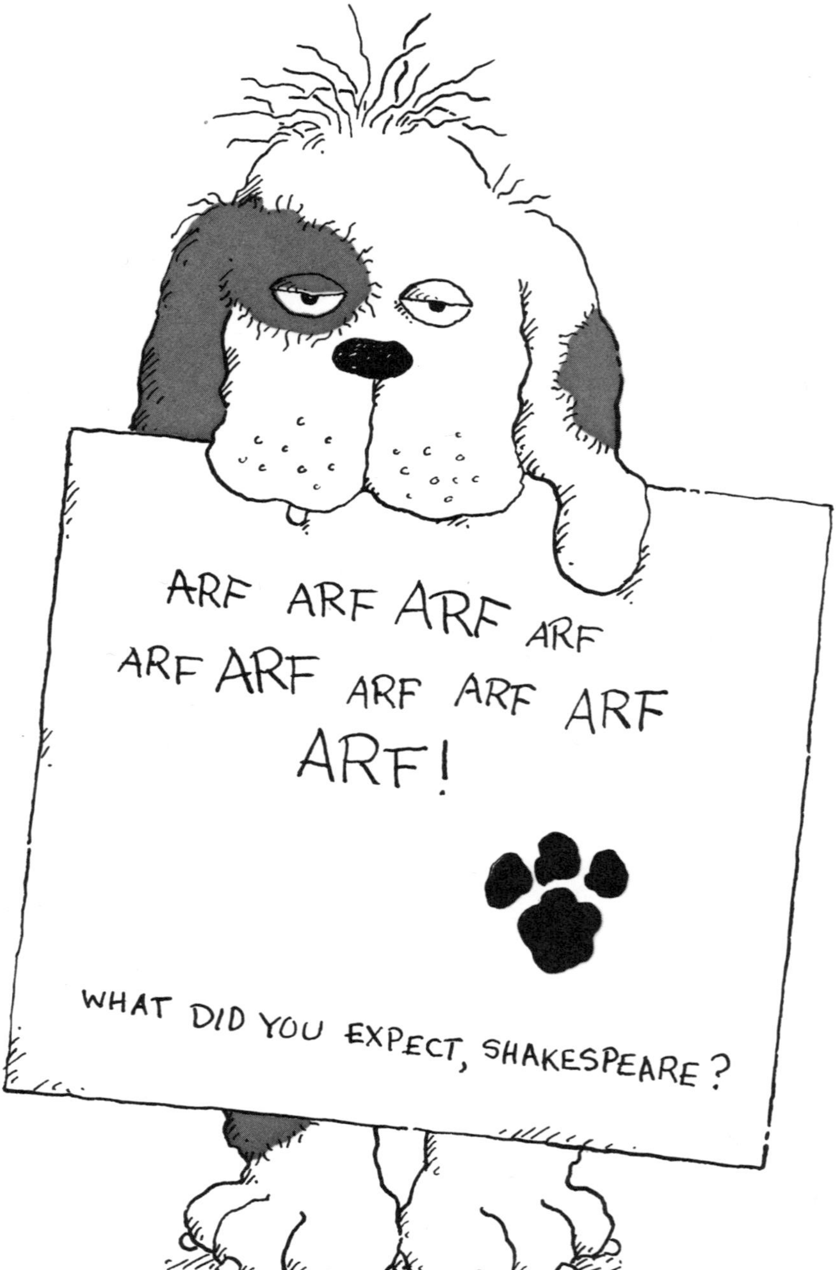
ARF ARF ARF ARF
ARF ARF ARF ARF ARF
ARF!
WHAT DID YOU EXPECT, SHAKESPEARE?

10 Things That *Won't* Make You Feel Better

1. Friends who bring you your homework so you won't miss too much while you're home.
2. Ice packs with sharp ice cubes inside.
3. Daytime TV shows in which almost every scene takes place in a hospital.
4. People who visit and tell you how much sicker *they* were when they had what you have.
5. Get well cards with angels on them.
6. People talking in whispers outside your bedroom door.
7. Brand-new pajamas that are so stiff, they crack when you bend your elbow.
8. A friend who calls to tell you not to worry about missing too much in school since they've spent the whole week getting ready for the Christmas party.
9. A doctor who begins your examination by asking if you're a boy or a girl.
10. Calling a friend and finding out that no one realized you'd been out for a week.

We interrupt this book to bring you this important information. . . .

10 Most Popular Medicines of the Middle Ages

1. Tree bark
2. Dry tree bark
3. Very dry tree bark
4. Slightly damp tree bark
5. Mostly wet tree bark
6. Damp tree bark that's been dried out
7. Slightly mildewed tree bark
8. Fast-acting tree bark with chlorophyll
9. Powdered dirt with tree bark mixed in
10. Children's-strength tree bark

Don't Just Lie There—Do Something (#2)

A Phoney Magic Trick
A Mind-Reading Trick You Can Learn

When you're sick, people are always trying to entertain you. Well, here's your chance to pull a switch and entertain them! In fact, you'll not only entertain them—you'll amaze and astound them with your mind-reading powers. All you need are a telephone, a friend, and a book that a friend also has. Here's the setup:

You call a friend on the phone and tell him or her that your illness has granted you secret powers, and that you can guess *any word* that he or she picks out of any book you both have a copy of! (One of your school textbooks is perfect for this.) Agree on which book you're going to use, and make sure you both have a copy in front of you. You'll both need a piece of paper and a pencil, too.

Now, tell your friend to open the book to any page, without telling you which page. Tell your friend to select any word on that page provided it is *in the first nine lines and within nine words of the left margin*. Make sure your friend understands that he or she must count lines from the top of the page and include chapter titles, captions, etc. And make sure your friend understands that he or she can select any one of the first nine words on any of the first nine lines, starting from the left side of the page.

Now, ask your friend to do the following arithmetic:

- Multiply the number of the page by 10.
- Add the number of the line to that total.
- Add 25.
- Multiply that sum by 10.
- Add the number of the word in the line. (For example, if your friend picked the fifth word from the left in that line, he or she would add 5.)

Ask your friend to give you the result. Let's say it's 2302. You are now ready to tell your friend the word he or she has selected. Here's how you do it:

Subtract 250 from the number your friend gave you. If the number is 2302, you subtract 250, and get 2052. The last digit of this number—2—is the number of the word. The next digit—5—is the number of the line. The remaining digits—20—are the page number.

Take your copy of the book, turn to page 20, count down to the fifth line, and find the second word in that line. Call it out loud and clear! We guarantee you'll be right.

Here's another example: Let's say your friend picks the fourth word in the fourth line of page 110. Here's how it would go. Your friend multiplies the page number by 10 ($110 \times 10 = 1100$). Then adds the number of the line ($1100 + 4 = 1104$). Then adds 25 ($1104 + 25 = 1129$). Then multiplies the sum by 10 ($1129 \times 10 = 11290$). Then adds the number of the word in the line ($11290 + 4 = 11294$).

Your friend tells you the number—11294. You quickly subtract 250 ($11294 - 250 = 11044$). You look at the number 11044. The last digit—4—is the number of the word. The next digit—4—is the number of the line. And the remaining digits—110—are the page number. Amazing!

20 Things You Can Do With Tissues

1. Stretch them out one by one to see how many tissues make a mile.
2. Hold one up to the sun and wait for an eclipse.
3. Glue 200 of them together to form a very light brick.
4. Wear white socks. Stuff them with 400 tissues. Ask people to sign your cast.
5. Sew different-colored tissues together to make a quilt for very hot nights.
6. Make confetti in case someone invites you to a New Year's Eve party.
7. Trade them with your friends until you've collected a complete set.
8. Send one to someone you don't like, and say that you've written a letter in invisible ink on it.
9. Knot 300 of them together and lower yourself out the window on them. (This one is only good if you weigh 8 pounds or less.)
10. Tell your friends you're giving them monogrammed handkerchief sets for Christmas this year. Then take out a bunch of tissues and write their initials on them with a felt-tip pen.
11. Stand on a box of tissues to see how you'll look when you're taller.
12. Roll several into small wads and paint them orange. Drop them into a bowl of water. Pretend you have goldfish.
13. Wear several of them in a stack on your head. See if anyone notices.
14. Dip 20 in water then watch to see which one dries first.
15. Roll 700,000 of them into a "snowman."

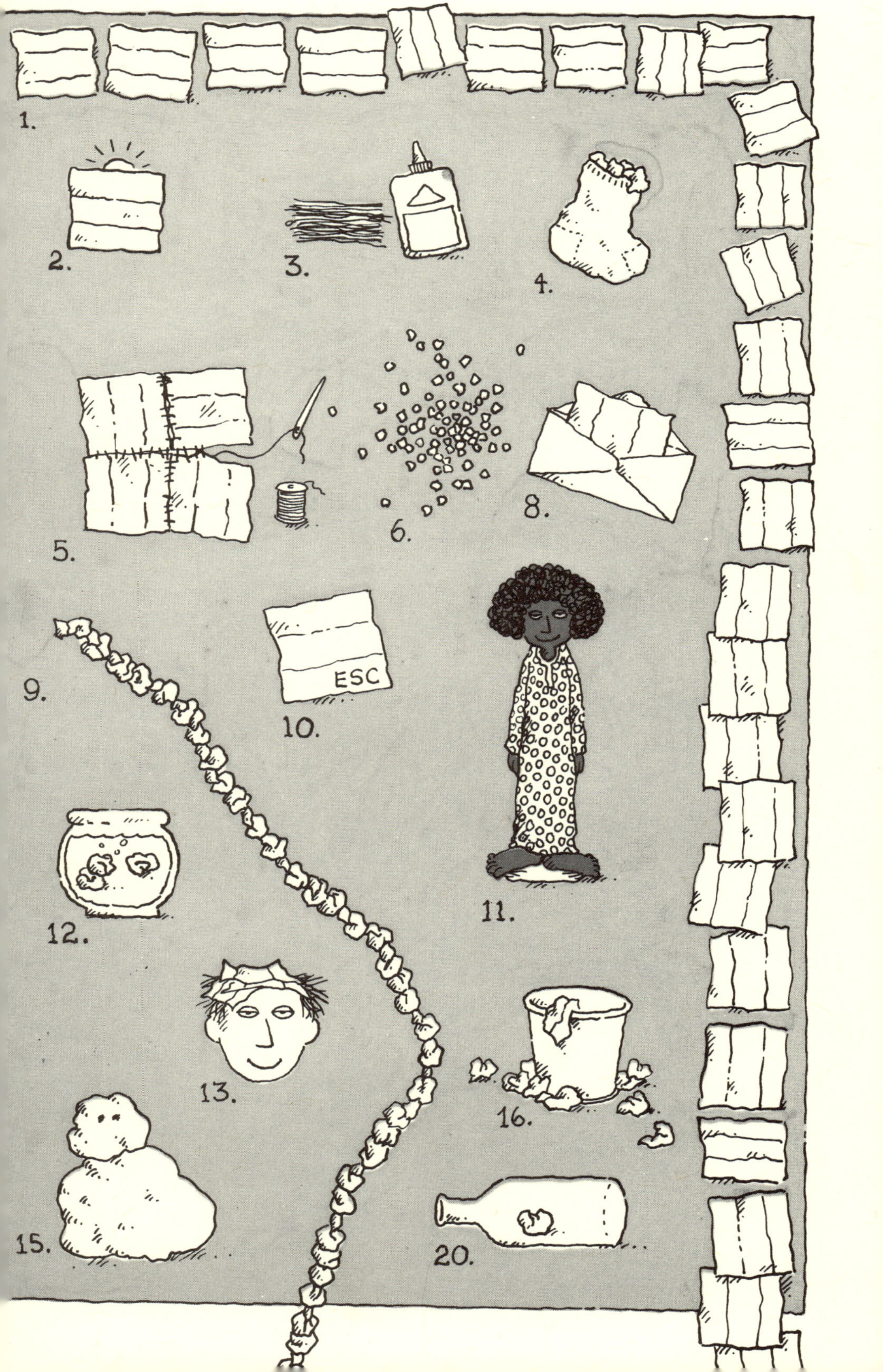
1.
2.
3.
4.
5.
6.
8.
9.
ESC
10.
11.
12.
13.
15.
16.
20.

16. See how many you can wad up and toss at the wastebasket across the room before someone asks you to stop.
17. Sew 400 of them together into a handy bag for keeping tissues in.
18. See if you can lift your weight in them.
19. Take 16 of them. Cut them into long strips and then fold them into quarters. Ask people to guess what you are making. When they give up, throw the tissues away.
20. Write messages on them and put them into bottles. Maybe some day you'll visit the ocean.

A Guide to Visitors

What They Say . . .
and What They Really Mean!

They say: Gee, you don't *look* sick!
They mean: You look *terrible!*

They say: Gosh, you look terrible!
They mean: Why did I come all the way over here? You don't even look sick!

They say: Everybody told me to send you their best wishes.
They mean: I couldn't get anyone else to come with me!

They say: Don't worry—you haven't missed much in school.
They mean: Unless you consider missing two world wars in history much!

They say: Did the doctor say there's a lot of what you've got going around?
They mean: Is it contagious? What am I doing here?!

They say: I'm sure you'll be up and about in no time.
They mean: Gee, you look *terrible!*

They say: Is there anything I can do for you?
They mean: I'd be glad to break in your brand-new bike or finish your lunch!

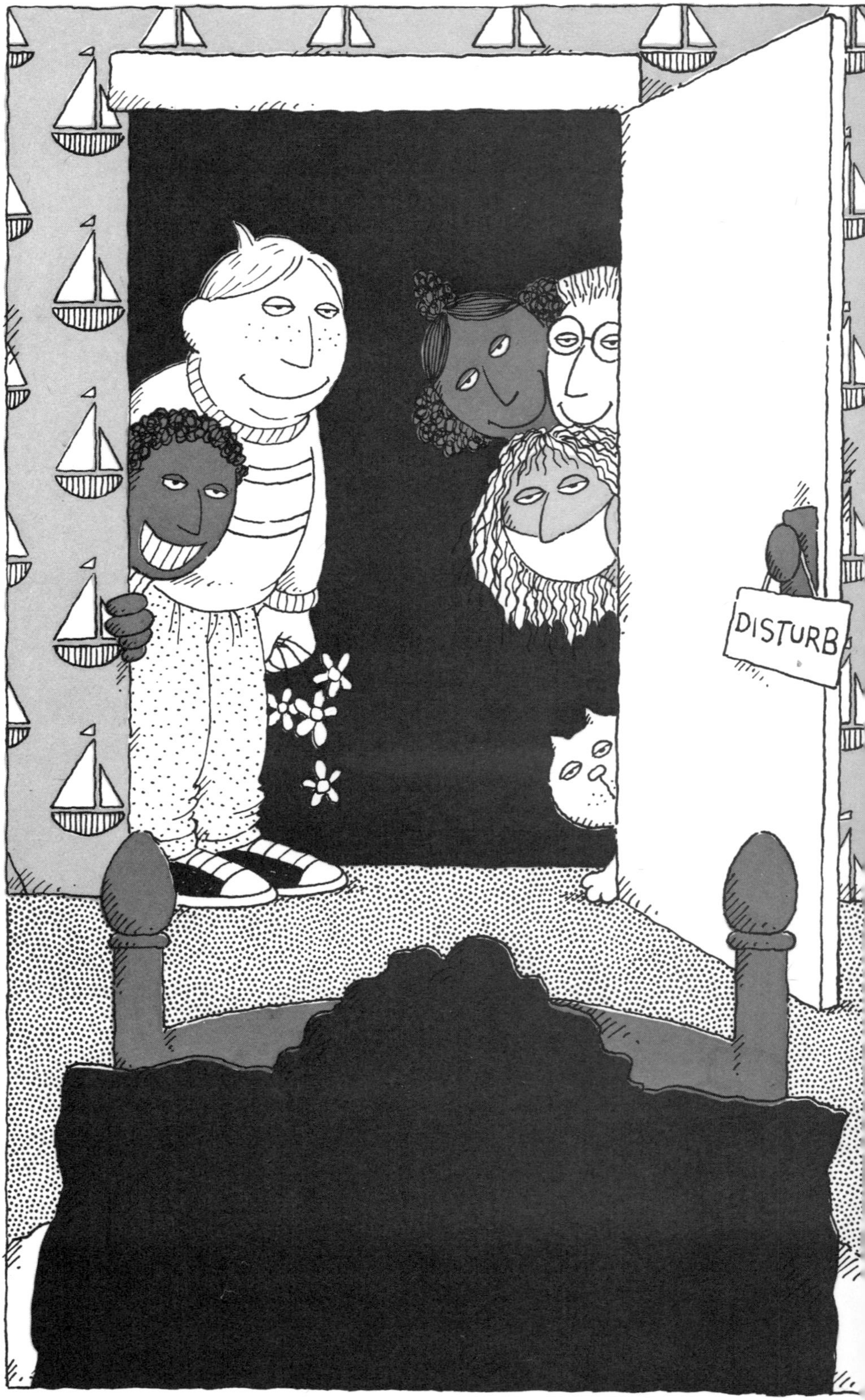
DISTURB

They say: Your mother said I can only stay a short time.
They mean: How long have I been sitting here—one year or two?

They say: Gee, what are all those different medicines for?
They mean: This ought to kill at least twenty minutes!

They say: The funniest thing happened in school today.
They mean: Nothing happened in school today, but anything's better than listening to a description of all your medicines!

They say: Well, I don't want to tire you out.
They mean: I can't wait to get out of here!

They say: Get well soon!
They mean: Because I'm not visiting again!

We interrupt this book to bring you this important advice. . . .

How To Tell an Antelope From a Moose

It's fairly easy to tell an antelope from a moose if you keep the following guidelines in mind:

Of the two, the antelope looks a lot more like an antelope than a moose. The moose, on the other hand, resembles the members of the moose family much more closely than those of the antelope family (if antelopes had families, which they don't).

Thank you.

Now, back to *The Sick of Being Sick Book*. . . .

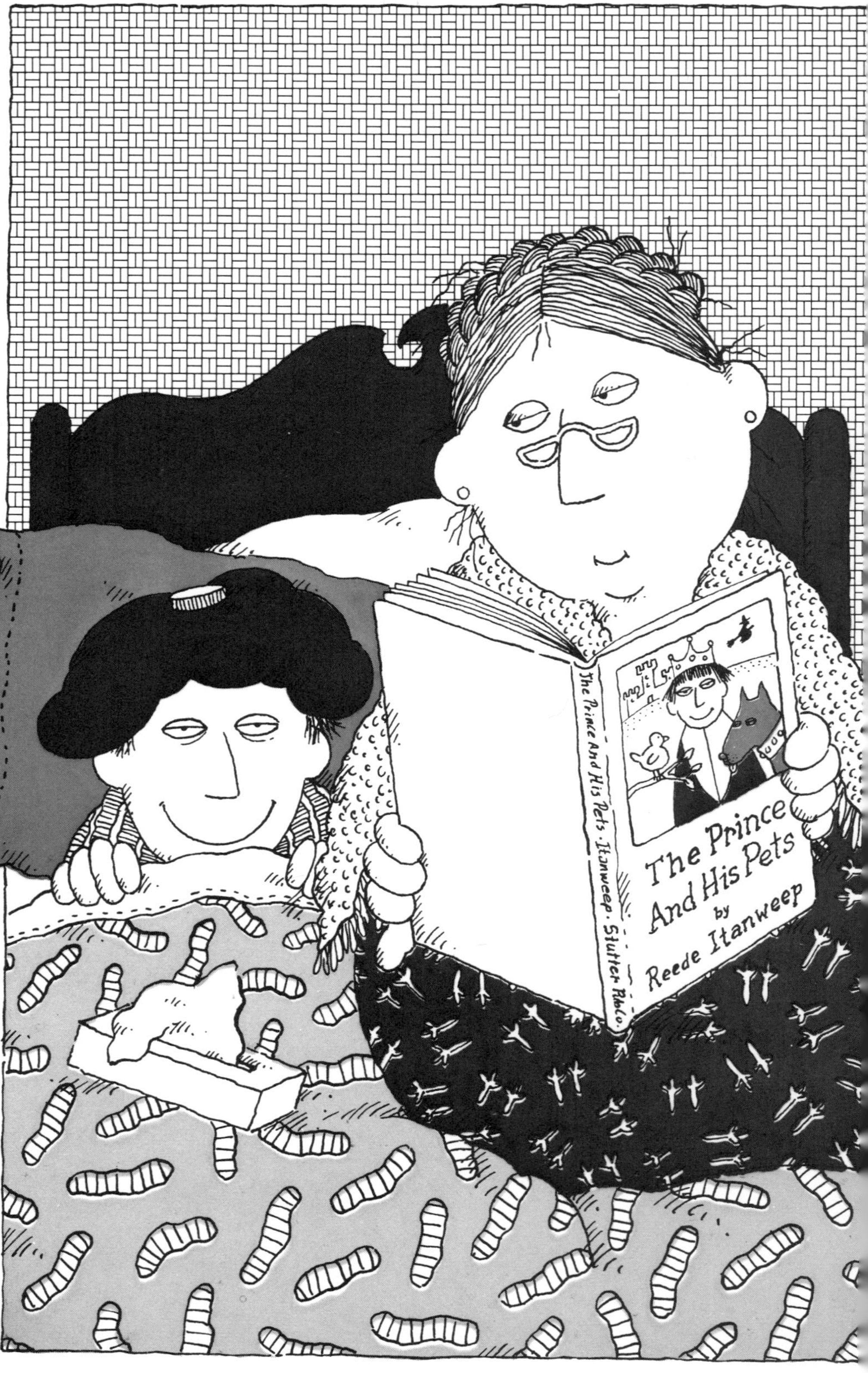
The Prince And His Pets
by
Reede Itanweep
The Prince And His Pets · Itanweep · Stutter Pkblc.

Read Me a Story!

A Joke To Play on an Eager Reader

When you're sick, someone always drags out an old storybook that you thought you had hidden away, and forces you to listen to some endless story about a debate between an ant and a grasshopper or a romance between a flower and a weed—stories no one would ever think of reading to a person who was well!

Well, here's your chance to have a little fun with that person in your family who's always dying to read to you when you're sick. Turn to the story on the next pages. Tell the Eager Reader that this is your favorite story in the whole world and beg to have it read to you.

Then lie back and try to keep a straight face.

THE PRINCE AND HIS PETS

by Reede Itanweep

Once upon a time there lived a handsome prince. His name was Prince Fitch Fission-Fashion the First.

Prince Fitch Fission-Fashion the First owned a French finch named Prince Fresh Finch and a Doberman pinscher named Pitch. Prince Fitch Fission-Fashion and Prince Fresh Finch, the prince's French finch, and the pinscher named Pitch were in a pinch. Fishing for hints, Prince Fitch Fission-Fashion winced.

Pitch itched. He may have had nits. "This is the pits!" cried Prince Fitch Fission-Fashion the First. "The prince's pinscher itching with nits! The pits! I suspect the witch. I sense her mitts in this sitch!"

Prince Fresh Finch, the dense French finch, was tense on his bench. To blitz the witch was no cinch. Not for a prince, a French finch named Prince Fresh Finch, and Pitch, a pinscher that itched. Pretending to seek fresh fish, the French finch flinched and minced to a niche in the ditch.

"He so scents a hitch, he's out of his wits!" complained Prince Fitch Fission-Fashion in a fit. With something amiss with Prince Fresh Finch, the missing French finch after fresh fish, Pitch itched without hitch. "Poor Pitch!"

Prince Fitch Fission-Fashion wished the witch the itch with which Pitch itched.

Prince Fitch Fission-Fashion the First inched over to Pitch, the pinscher who itched, and gave him a pinch which gave the prince hints, for he saw French finch prints on Pitch. "It was no witch which gave nits to itch Pitch!" cried Prince Fitch Fission-Fashion the First. "There are hints of French finch prints; hence the nits that itch Pitch come from Prince Fresh Finch, the French finch amiss after fresh fish in the niche in the ditch!"

"No need to lynch!" cried Prince Fresh Finch, the French finch tense in the trench. He used a winch to pinch out of the ditch, saying, "Perhaps I'm a dunce, but the deep tints and dense scents from the pinscher Pitch are hints he should rinse!"

"Rinse!" cried Prince Fitch Fission-Fashion, sensing his mission. "Itch—hence rinse!"

Pitch, the itching pinscher, flinched, winced—then washed. Then, Prince Fitch Fission-Fashion the First called, "Here, Prince! Here, Prince Fresh Finch!" No dunce, the French finch needed no hints to rinse.

In a pinch, the rinse rid the French finch and the itching pinscher of the itch and the nits, and the Prince (Fitch Fission-Fashion), the French finch (Prince Fresh Finch), and the pinscher (the itchless Pitch) lived happily ever since.

"There's a Lot of That Going Around. . . ."

Is the conversation in your sickroom getting a little dull? Don't worry—*The Sick of Being Sick Book* is here to give you a new outlook on all the tired old phrases you've been hearing ever since you sneezed your first sneeze. How? Well, have you ever pictured in your mind what the following phrases really mean? We did—and we found they can be a lot more fun if you . . .

Get the Picture!

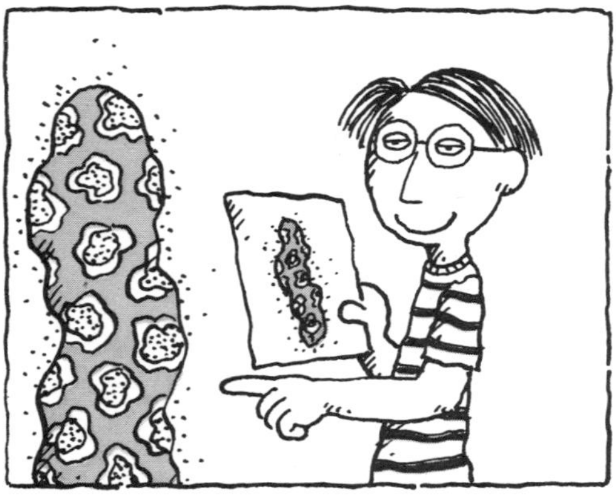

RECOGNIZING A SYMPTOM

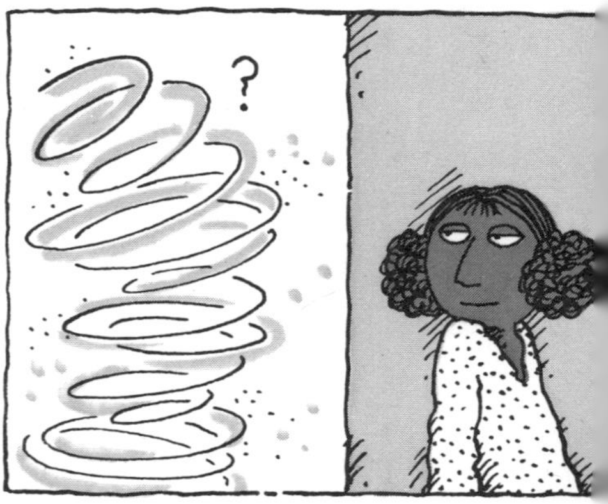

AVOIDING A DRAFT

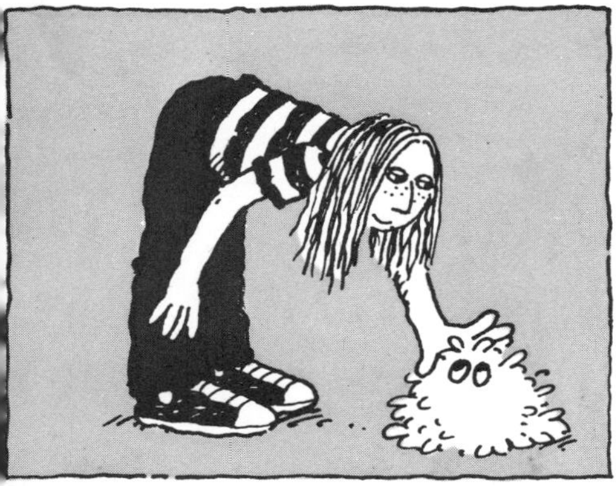

FEELING A LITTLE WOOZY

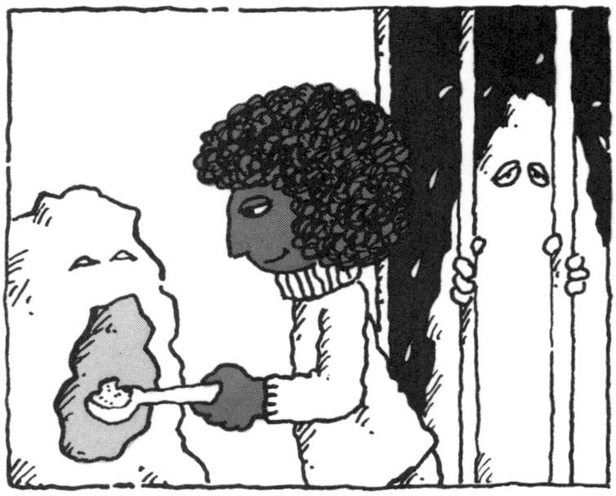

FEEDING A COLD AND STARVING A FEVER

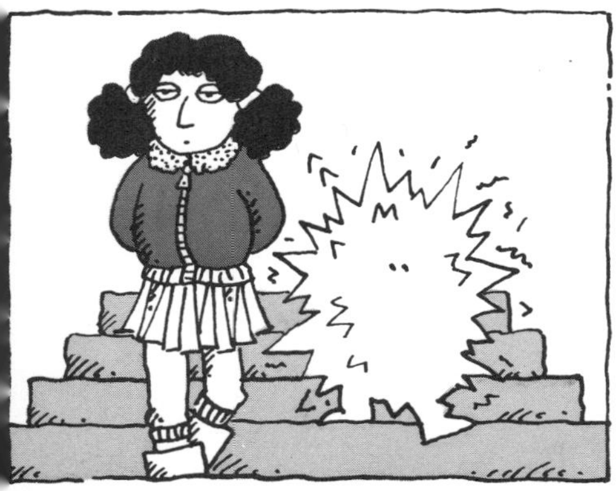

COMING DOWN WITH A CHILL

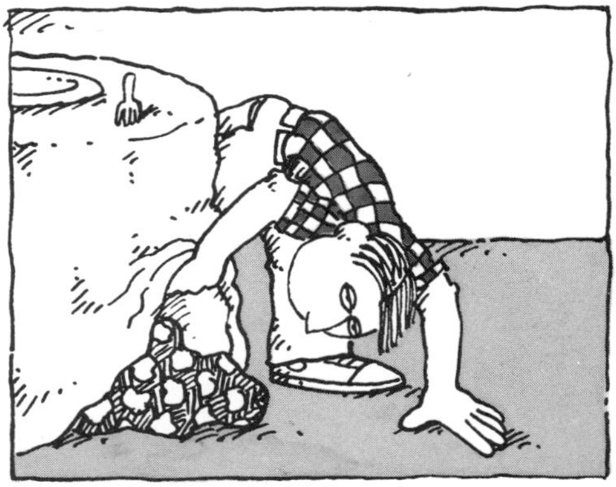

LOSING YOUR APPETITE

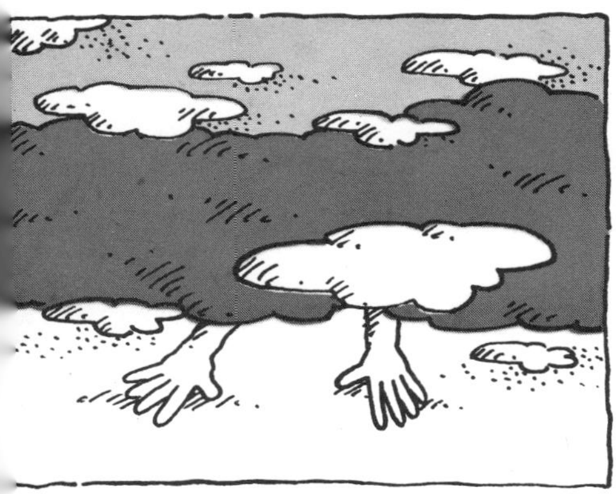

FEELING UNDER THE WEATHER

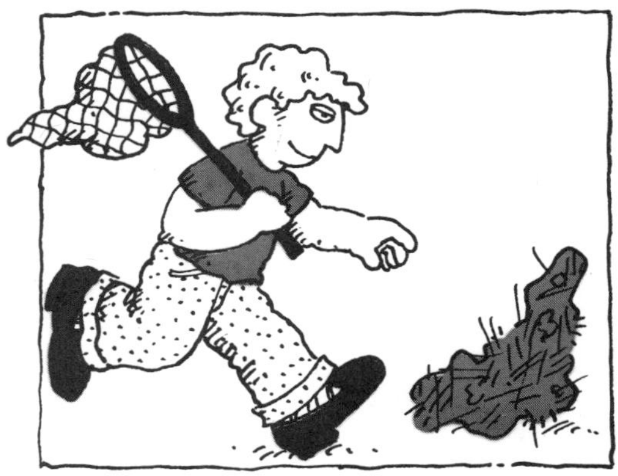

CATCHING A VIRUS

Don't Just Lie There—
Do Something (#3)

Drop-A-Line Code
How To Send Secret Messages

Do you realize what has happened to your friends while you've been sick? The poor unfortunates have been deprived of your sparkling personality and wit! The least you can do is drop them a note and help them through these dark days without you.

But don't help them too much. Why shouldn't they work a little to figure out what you're up to? Write your messages in *The Sick of Being Sick Book* secret way, and they'll be cracking up before they can crack your code!

The Drop-A-Line Code is very easy to learn—but oh-so-hard to decipher—unless you know the secret. Check out the message at the top of the next page.

↓ ↓

WDOGROOTYOIPRSUWALLDFREBPLOOFGBMIP
HOOPLADFREAGJOOLLLKMNUIEPOOGHIOPRT
TREEAPLINTMOLKGHUJIKIOKIMNRDFERTVW
BBBREATGHUSHHHRRRRTTTCCNUUUIIPPYUR
FFFFRRRREEIJJJJCDEFGHUIGFRUYVTERDF
HTYUFGTHYCCCGHJKLMNOPRTSDEFGRTFDER
BYUIOBYUIOKBYUIOPBYUIOPIBYUIOPBYUI
DERFGDERFGODFREGDFREGDFCGHYUIDFRGH
CVGRTCVRGTFCVRGTCVRGTCVKGTYUIGTUIB

The message above actually says, I AM SICK OF BEING SICK. Here's how it works: Take a sheet of paper and fold it in thirds the long way. The paper now has two long vertical creases.

Now, write your message down along the creases. Once your message is complete, fill up the rest of the space with nonsense syllables, confused letters, or anything you want.

After your friends drive themselves nuts for a while, you can let them in on the secret. When they read down the folds, your message will be clear. Give it a try—it'll surely put a new wrinkle in your writing!

How To Survive Daytime Television

We all know that being sick means you must watch hour after hour of daytime TV. But there's one problem—after a while, all those silly game shows, ancient reruns of old comedy shows, kiddie programs, and slow-moving soap operas can begin to make you sicker than you were before you turned on the set!

So take a break, turn off the television set, and read *our* version of daytime TV. Instead of groaning, you'll be laughing. And you won't have to keep getting up every five minutes.—We'll change the channel for you. . . .

CLICK!

"All right, Mrs. Treeblight, you've already won a mohair camper, a set of red, white, and blue chimney logs, a fur bowling ball, a new all-vinyl wardrobe for yourself and your entire family, and the keys to the vault at the First Bank of Sydney, Australia! Do you want to stop here—or do you want to go on to Round Three?"

"GO ON! GO ON!" "GO HOME! GO HOME!" "TAKE THE PRIZES!" "TAKE A CHANCE!" "TAKE A WALK!"

"Please, audience—no coaching! Which will it be, Mrs. Treeblight—the prizes? Or a chance for a three-year trip to the planet of your choice by going on to Round Three?"

"I—I can't decide, Don. I just can't decide. Can I come back tomorrow and tell you my decision?"

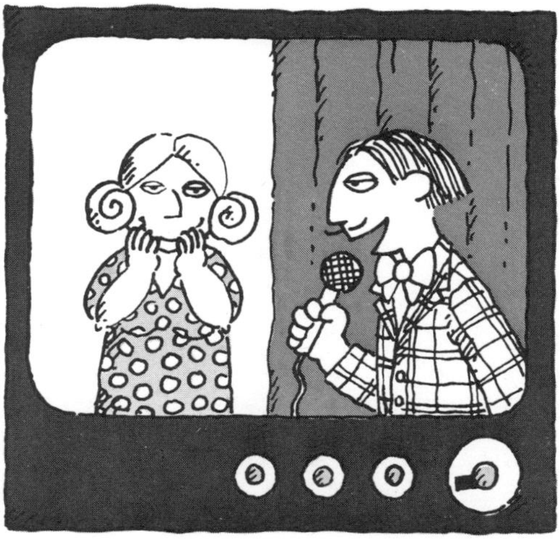

CLICK!

"I—I can't decide, Marcia. You know I like staying here with you, playing Parcheesi on your rented card table. But what about Doris and her knees?"

"Her knees, Martin? What about Doris's knees? Please—you must tell me. I *must know!*"

"It isn't pleasant, Marcia. That's why I treasure these moments here with you, these moments we spend around your rented card table. Doris's knees . . . well . . . ever since the accident, they—"

"Yes, yes—go on Martin. You must tell me—you must!"

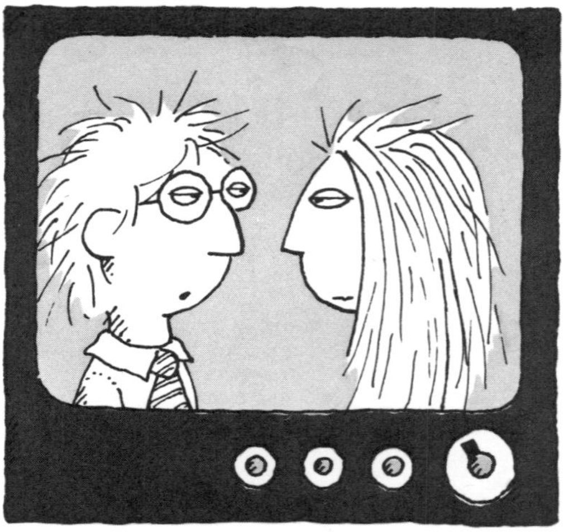

"Marcia, it's so painful to tell. But I'll try. I'll try. Doris's knees . . . they have little faces painted on them. Little eyes . . . a little nose . . . a big red smile. A face on each knee. I don't know how they got there. Sometimes I think I might be . . . losing my mind!"

"Martin, how awful for you—"

CLICK!

"Lucy, how awful for you! You've been locked in the closet all day with ten pounds of pastry dough rising on your face?"

"That's right, Ricky. I was afraid to call for help. I didn't want the dough to fall!"

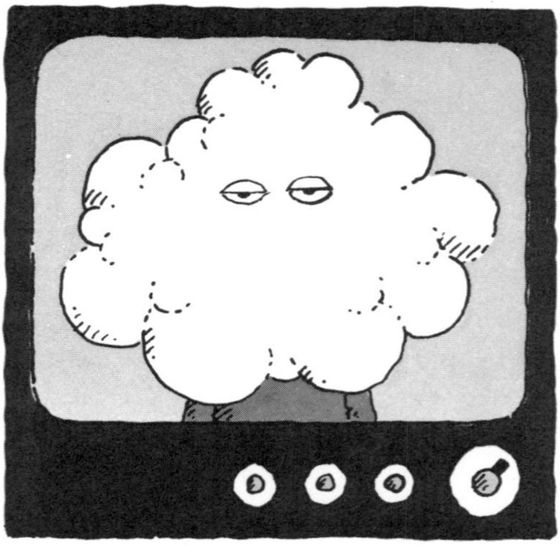

CLICK!

"That's right, Mrs. Roachspray—let it fall! Let it fall! You need six more drops to beat the other couple!"

"I think I can do it, Bud!"

"If you do, Mrs. Roachspray, you win an all-expense-paid vacation in the underwater log cabin of your choice! Come on, let it fall!"

"It's . . . it's falling, Bud!"

"Yes . . . yes, it is! SHE DID IT! SHE DID IT, AUDIENCE! SHE DROPPED THE CABBAGE!"

"YAAAAAAAAAAY!"

"You've shown them how it's done, Mrs. Roachspray! Way to go! That's the way we play the sensational, new fun game, 'Drop That Cabbage!'"

YAAAAAAAAAAAAAAAAAAAAY!

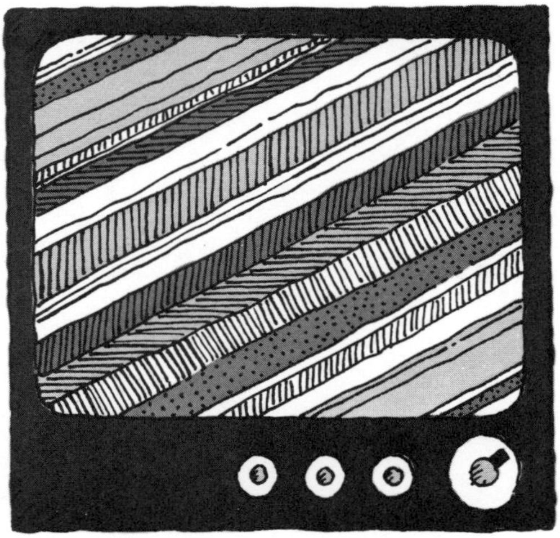

CLICK!

"AAAAAAAAAAY!"

"Stop crying, Lucy. Fred and I will get all this shoe polish off your face before Ricky gets home."

CLICK!

"Big Weasel, get away from that chicken coop! Big Weasel, come over here and show the boys and girls how to write the number *4*. Big Weasel, come back here! Put that chicken down! What about the number *4*, Big Weasel? Show them how— Stop him! Stop him! He's eating that chicken! Big Weasel, this is disgusting! You're supposed to be cute and lovable! You're not supposed to tear off a chicken's head and—"

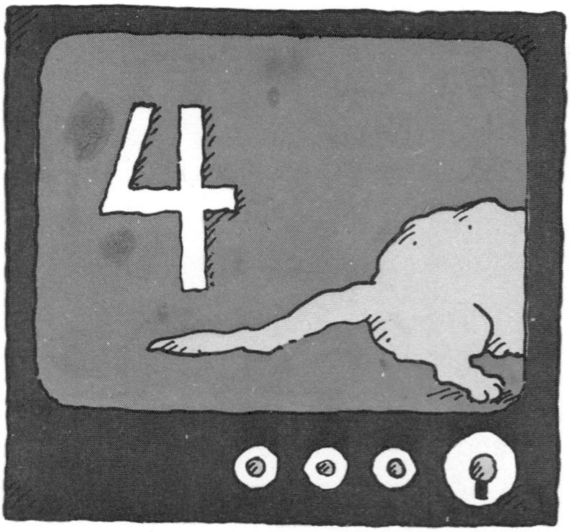

CLICK!

"Marjorie, what are you crying about? Is it me? Is it my torn shirt? Please don't cry because I tore my shirt. You know that I always tear my shirts. It's one of the things you used to love about me. Remember the day we met? You were walking to the post office to mail your grandfather to Cleveland. You stopped when you saw that I had my arm caught in a mailbox. I'll never forget that tender look on

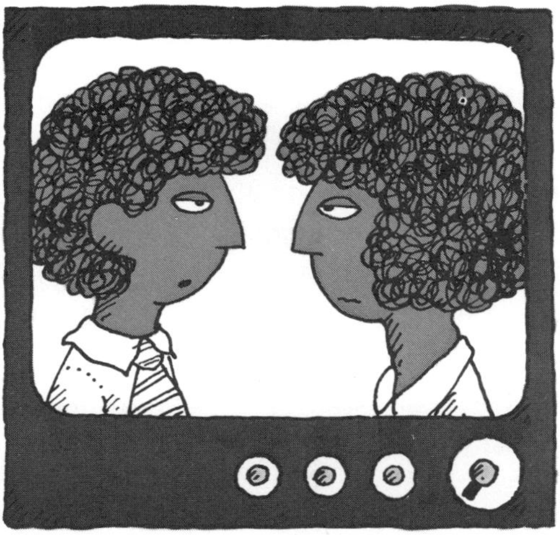

your face, that look that seemed to say, 'Why does he have his arm caught in a mailbox?'

"I tore my shirt that day, too, Marjorie. Remember? Of course you do. That's why you're crying now, isn't it?"

"Norman, you *know* I always cry when I chop onions!"

CLICK!

"—That's right, you can buy two hundred pounds of chopped onions for the price of a hundred ninety-nine pounds of chopped onions when you shop at Shop & Chop, where we chop our food *up* so we can chop prices *down*! Now, let's get back to our 'Midday Movie Matinee in the Morning,' *Seasick in Kansas*, starring Parsley Sage and Rosemary N. Thyme."

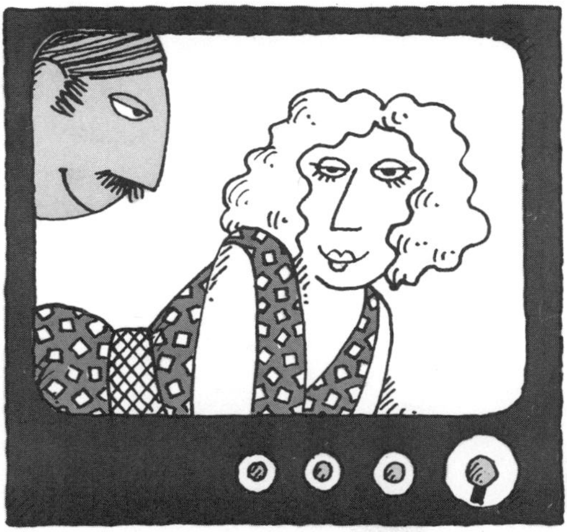

CLICK!

"—Two hundred pounds of chopped onions, the ocean liner of your choice, a year's supply of murky bilge water—and that's not all you can win on 'Choose Your Choice!' Tell them what else they can win, Don Bardo!"

"Thirty plastic bags filled with moist cat food, a matching set of electric cattle prods, a gold earmuff, steam-operated crabgrass tweezers in a handy carrying case, and that's not all! Tell them what else they can win, Bud LeBeau!"

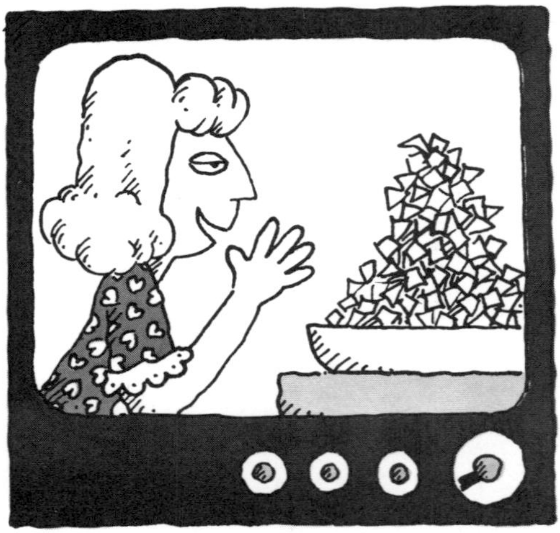

"A carton of no-smudge, no-stick elephant remover, a mix-and-match set of double-lined trash bags in the color of your choice, a sterling-silver wild-goose caller, a set of plastic bunk beds for gerbils—and that's not all you can win on 'Choose Your Choice!' Tell them what else they can win, Eddie Sparks!"

"A set of matched—"

CLICK!

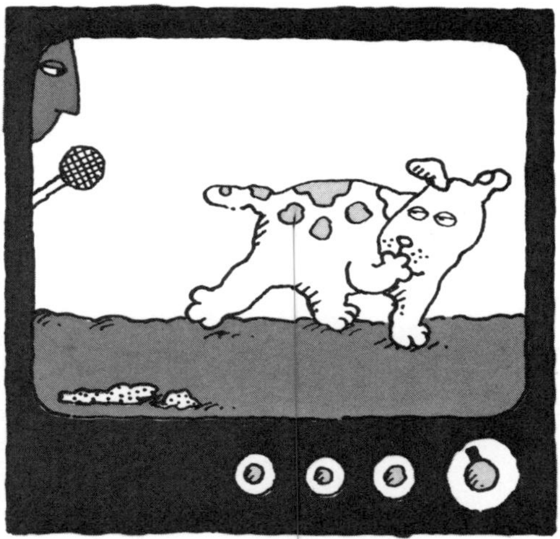

"A dog became violently ill on Main Street this morning, and "Midday News" reporter Gloria Hallelujah was there to cover the story. Gloria, what's the situation on Main Street at this moment?"

CLICK!

"But, Lucy, you can't hide those ten puppies from Ricky forever! What if he wants to take a bath? He's sure to see them when he runs his bathwater!"

"But, Ethel—I promised I'd take care of the puppies for twelve years until the owners get back!"

CLICK!

"Well, Mr. and Mrs. Bathwater, it's a pleasure to welcome you as contestants on 'Make It or Fake It!'"

"Thank you, Bud. It's a pleasure being here."

"Now, you're familiar with the rules of our game, aren't you?"

"Well, no, actually we're not. We've never seen the show before."

"You don't know how to play our game?"

"No. No, we don't. I'm afraid you'll have to explain the rules to us."

"Well . . . I'm new to the show myself. I was the host on 'Dialing for Cotton Balls' until it went off the air last week. So I'm really not too certain of the rules myself. Gee, perhaps *you* can tell our contestants how we play 'Make It or Fake It,' announcer Jack Bando."

"I've been announcer on this show for three years, Bud, and I *still* can't figure out how the game is played!"

"How about our studio audience? Does anyone here know how to play this game? Anyone at all? Come on—someone must know the rules! Doesn't anyone—"

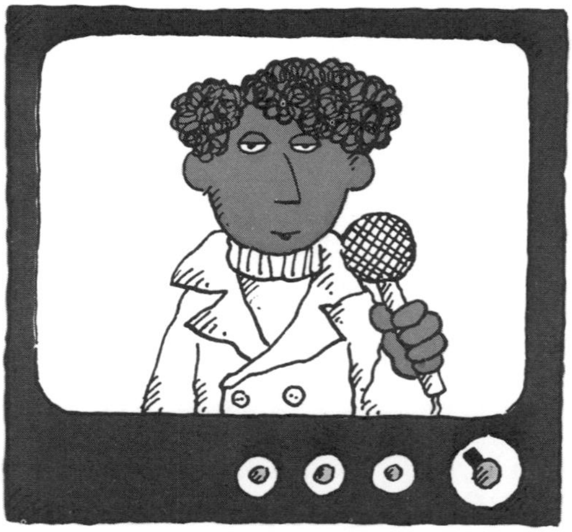

CLICK!

"—And that's the news. Turning to the weather for the tri-state area . . . Partly cloudy this afternoon, with a tornado moving in by evening, followed by earthquakes, a

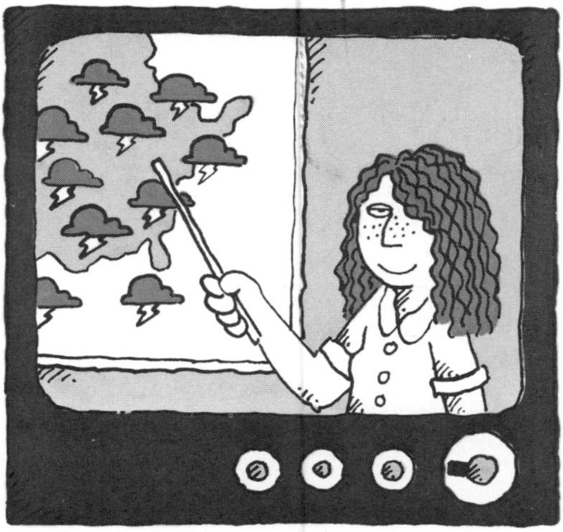

monsoon, and a giant tidal wave that will wipe the entire area off the face of the earth by tonight. More details on the 'Eleven O'clock News'. . . ."

CLICK!

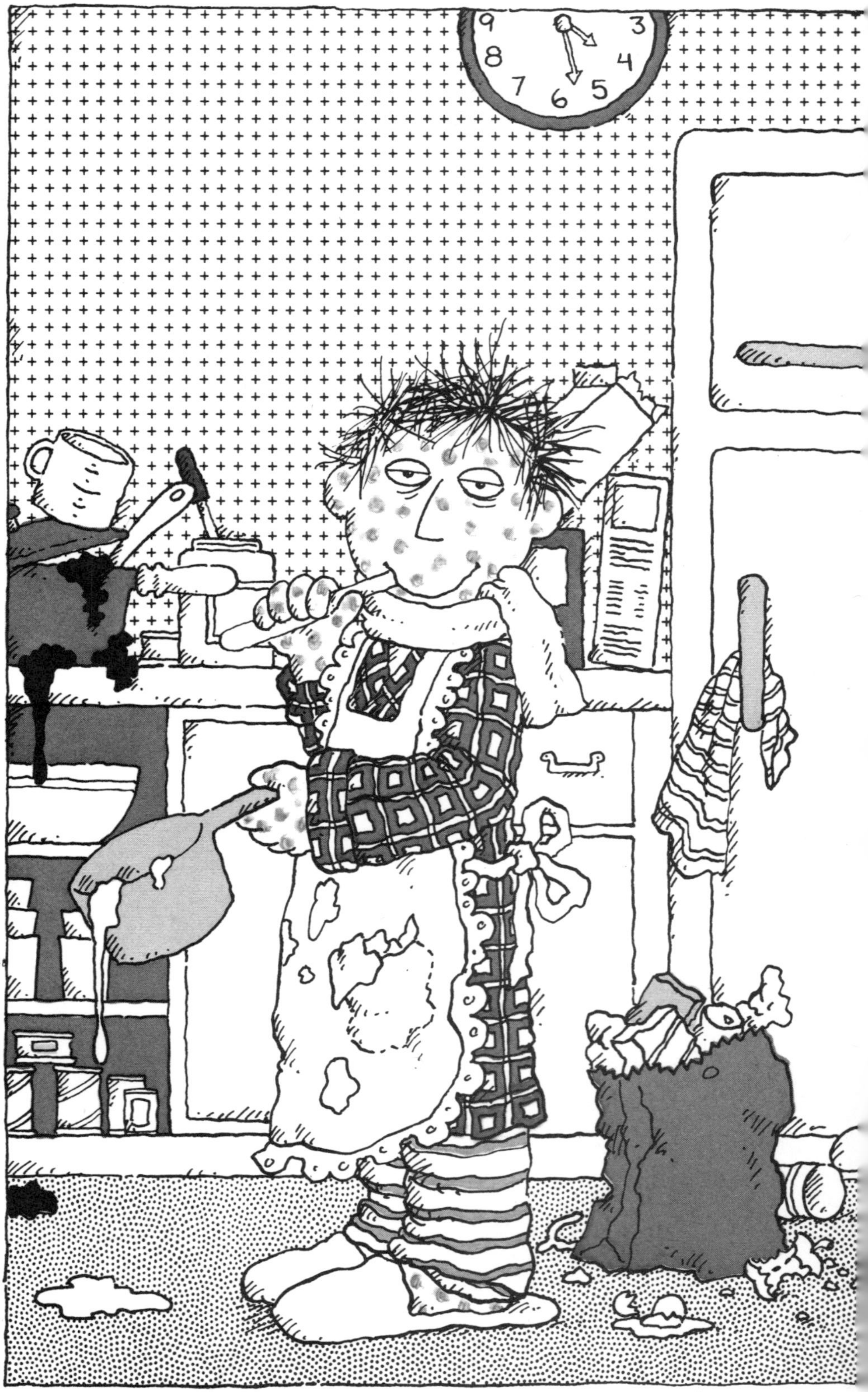

Warmer-uppers, Cooler-offers, and Tasty Treat-ments

Bored with tea and toast? Well, try tea and toast—but try them our way! Here are some new recipe ideas for unbeatable eatables that are bound to beat the bed-tray blahs. All of these recipes are easy to swallow—and a cinch to follow. So if the doctor and the chief of the kitchen agree, you can make them yourself. Or, if you prefer, let others do the mixing, the stirring, and the cooking, while you save your strength for the really important job—the eating!

WARMER-UPPERS

Glass Sipper

This recipe comes to you from Russia with love. You'll need:

1 tall thick glass (an ice-cream-soda glass, if possible)
boiling water
1 tea bag
raspberry jam (or any other flavor you like)
a long spoon

Make the tea in the glass. Add a spoonful of jam, and stir with the long spoon. Sip the tea slowly, adding more jam if you wish.

Tea-rific Treat

Sweeten up your tea with a naturally delicious treat at the bottom. You'll need:

1 round slice of orange
2 teaspoons of honey
a dash of cinnamon
boiling water
1 tea bag
milk

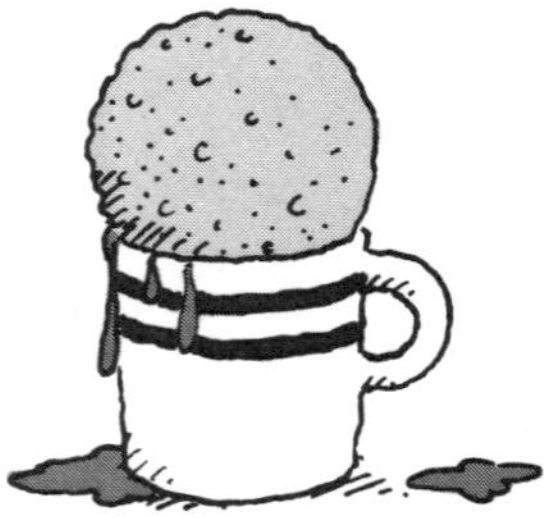

Put a round orange slice in the bottom of a mug or cup. Spoon the honey over it, and sprinkle it with cinnamon. Fill the cup with boiling water (leave a little room for milk). Dunk the tea bag into the water until the tea is dark enough. Add a splash of milk, and stir.

When you've finished the tea, eat the honey-drenched orange slice for a supersweet ending.

Great Grape Grog

Add a little spice to your life with this warming drink. You'll need:

1 cup of grape juice
a cinnamon stick
(or ¼ teaspoon of powdered cinnamon)
2 cloves
a dash of nutmeg
a dash of ginger
a slice of lemon
a small saucepan or pot
a long spoon for stirring

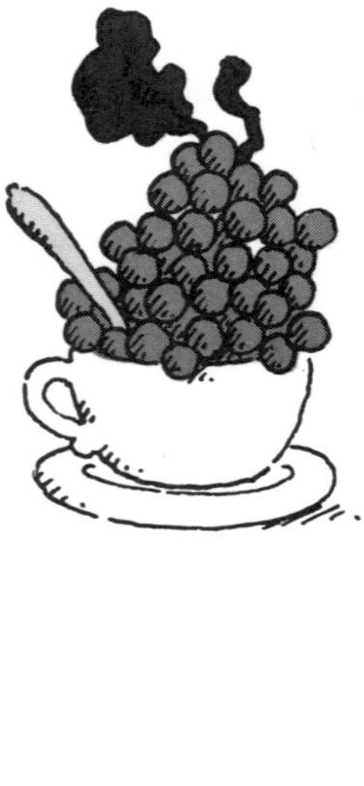

Put everything except the lemon slice in the pot or saucepan. Put the pot on very low heat, and stir the liquid a few times while it's warming. Don't let the mixture bubble up and boil—just warm it. Pour the grog into a mug or cup. Top it off with the lemon slice, and drink.

Souper Bowl Team-Up

Who says soup has to be dull? Try it with a hot crust baked right on the bowl! You'll need:

an ovenproof soup bowl or mug
any kind of soup
a paper towel
butter or margarine
prepared crescent-roll dough that comes in a tube
pot holders or oven mitts

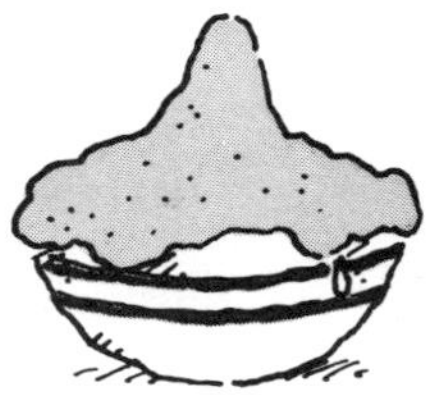

First of all, make sure that your soup bowl or mug is ovenproof. Check it out with the keeper of the kitchen before you do anything else. Then make sure you've got the right kind of rolls. You need the kind that you roll up yourself and then bake.

Okay? Ready to begin. Preheat the oven to the temperature suggested on the dough package. Fill your ovenproof bowl or mug with warm soup. Put a little butter or margarine on a paper towel and grease the rim of the bowl or mug. Take one or two of the triangular pieces of dough out of the tube and press them around the rim of the bowl or mug. You'll probably need two triangles to go all the way around a bowl, one triangle for a mug.

Put the bowl or mug in the oven. In about ten minutes, your soup will be surrounded by a golden brown, delicious crust. Using pot holders or mitts, take the bowl or mug out of the oven. Let it cool a little, and then dig in!

Thirst Ade Kit

When you're really thirsty, your body needs salt. Here's a delicious way to get that salt. You'll need:

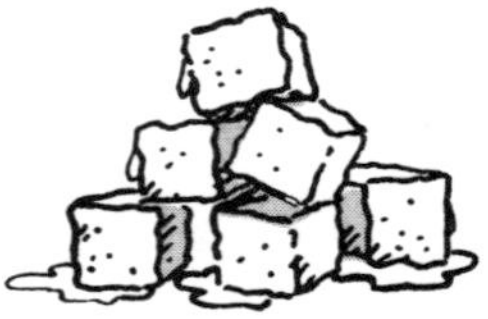

1 ice-cube tray
2 cups of canned pineapple juice
1 tall glass
Gatorade

This takes a little preparation, but it's worth it. Fill an empty ice-cube tray with pineapple juice. Let the juice freeze until you have pineapple-juice ice cubes. Put a couple of cubes in a tall glass (leave the rest in the freezer to use later). Then fill the glass with Gatorade. (Gatorade is loaded with salt, but it tastes sweet.) Drink slowly. This is one drink that will never get that watery, been-sitting-around-all-day taste. As the cubes melt, the drink gets more and more pineapple-y and more delicious.

(If you don't like pineapple juice, any other flavor of juice will do.)

Ice And Easy Fruit Punch

Another cool ice-cube trick. You'll need:

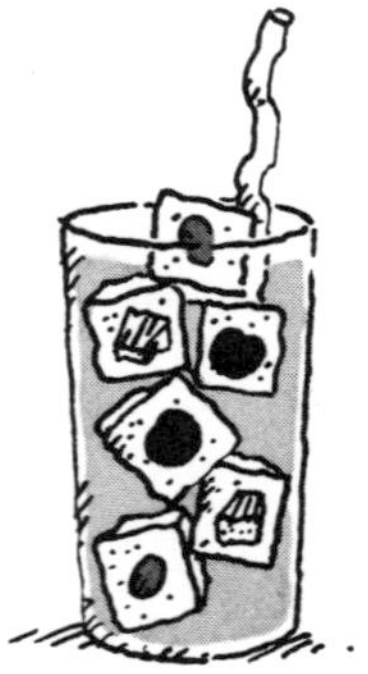

1 ice-cube tray
1 cup of canned fruit cocktail
water
a tall glass
1 cup of orange juice
ginger ale

Put the fruit cocktail in the ice-cube tray. Add water until the tray is full. Move the fruit around so there's fruit in every section of the tray. Freeze into cubes.

Put several of your fruit-filled cubes into a tall glass. Add the orange juice. Fill the rest of the glass with ginger ale. Stir and sip. When the cubes melt, eat the fruit.

Strawberry Short Shake

This recipe makes enough for 3 or 4 shakes. You can store what's left over in the refrigerator. You'll need:

an electric blender
1 small package of frozen strawberries
3 cups of milk
1 drop of red food coloring

Put the berries in the blender. Add the milk and the food coloring, and turn on the blender. (Make sure the top is on first!) The shake is ready when everything appears to be mixed together smoothly.

Purple Punch And Munch More

This drink-and-snack tastes better if you make a whole pitcher at a time. Store what's left over in the refrigerator. You'll need:

a pitcher (It should hold 2 quarts.)
1 orange
1 lemon
1 apple
a small can of pineapple chunks
1 quart of grape juice
club soda

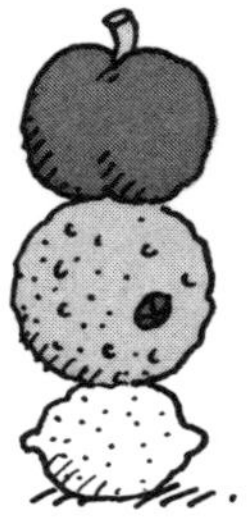

Slice up the orange, lemon, and apple, and drop all the slices into the bottom of the pitcher. Add the pineapple chunks. Add the grape juice. Let the mixture sit for a couple of hours in the refrigerator.

Put a couple of spoonfuls of the fruit in a glass, and then fill the glass with the juice. Leave a little room for a splash of club soda. Drink the punch and then munch the fruit!

TASTY TREAT-MENTS

Bread Winners

Add the artistic touch to toast for a tasty change. You'll need:

bread (white or whole wheat)
cookie cutters
your choice of:
- butter or margarine
- cottage cheese
- cinnamon sugar
- apple and orange slices
- jam
- multicolored sprinkles
- American cheese

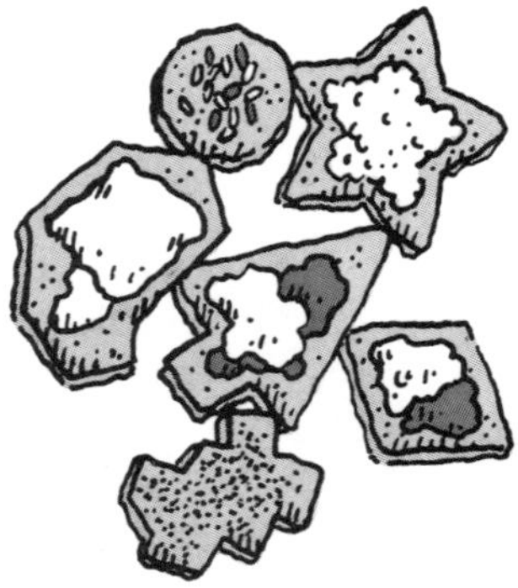

Why does toast have to be square? Use cookie cutters to cut your bread into more interesting shapes. If you don't have any cookie cutters, use a glass to make nice even circles—or use a knife to cut out hearts, triangles, or diamonds. When you've got your bread shapes all cut out, you're ready to try the following treats:

- Spread jam and cottage cheese on a bread shape. Top with colored sprinkles. Toast in a toaster-oven or broiler for a few minutes.
- Spread butter or margarine on bread shapes. Sprinkle on cinnamon sugar. Toast under a broiler until brown.
- Put a thin slice of apple on a bread shape. Top with a slice of American cheese. Toast under a broiler until the cheese melts.
- Spread butter or margarine on a bread shape. Place a thin slice of orange on top, and sprinkle the orange with cinnamon. Toast under a broiler until brown.

Now, make up your own combinations!

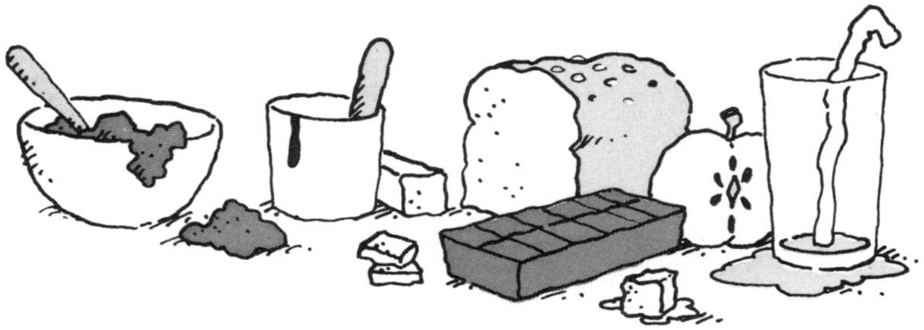

Applesauce-ery

To make this applesauce with a difference, you'll need:

1 cup of applesauce
1 cup of cranberry sauce
a dash of ginger

Mix the applesauce and the cranberry sauce together. Add a dash of ginger. Chill the mixture in the refrigerator until you're ready to eat it. This recipe makes 4 servings. Store what's left over in the refrigerator.

Crunch-A-Bunch

To make the world's simplest snack food—frozen grapes—you'll need:

grapes, separated
into small bunches
small plastic bags

Put each bunch of grapes into an individual plastic bag. Place the bags in the freezer for several hours. Then, when you feel like having something cool to suck on, take out one bag of grapes at a time. Pop the frozen grapes into your mouth like candy!

Cook-A-Noodle-Do

This noodle pudding tastes so good, it's hard to believe it's good for you—but it is! You'll need:

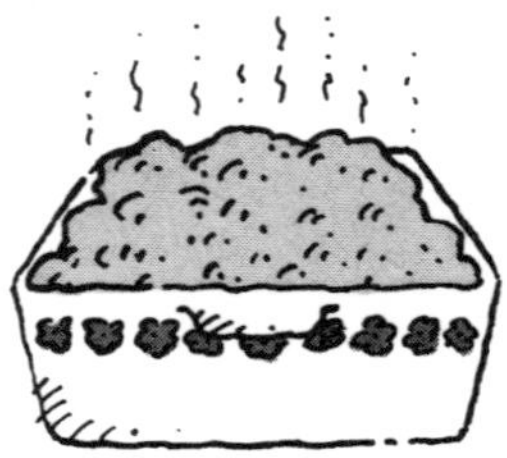

- 2 cups of cooked noodles
- butter or margarine
- a paper towel
- an ovenproof casserole or baking dish
- 1 egg
- a mixing bowl
- ½ cup of milk
- a fork
- 1½ cups of cottage cheese
- 3 tablespoons of sugar
- ½ cup of raisins
- cinnamon

First, con someone into cooking the noodles for you—or cook them yourself by following the directions on the noodle package. Use about one cup of uncooked noodles to get the right amount of cooked noodles.

Preheat the oven to 375°F. Put a small amount of butter or margarine on a paper towel, and grease the casserole or baking dish. Break the egg into the mixing bowl, add the milk, and beat them together with a fork until you have a nice, light yellow mixture. Now add the cottage cheese, sugar, and noodles. Stir until everything looks mixed together. Stir in the raisins. Then pour the whole mixture into the casserole or baking dish. Sprinkle with cinnamon.

Bake at 375°F. for about 45 minutes. Makes 4 servings. Eat it warm or cold.

We interrupt this book to bring you this important advice. . . .

8 Tips for Bathing an Angry Rhinoceros

1. Be careful.
2. Take care.
3. Be very careful.
4. Be as careful as you can.
5. Use extreme caution and care.
6. Proceed carefully.
7. Try to make sure the water isn't too hot.
8. Don't tickle.

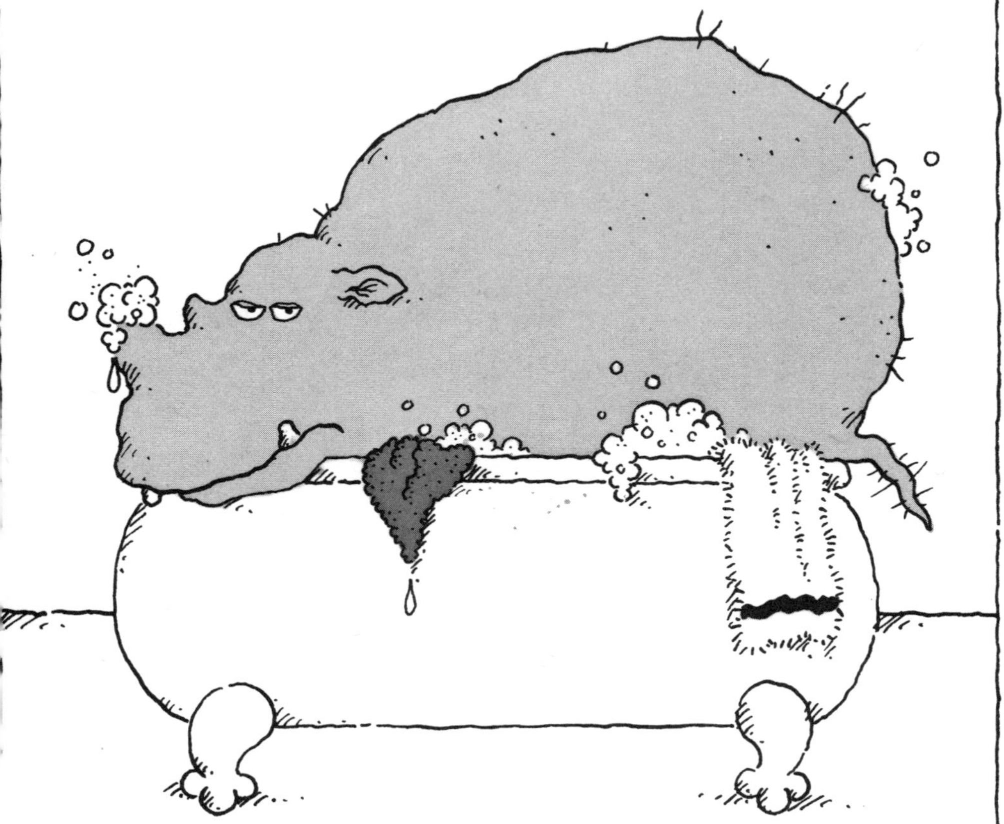

Here they are, those award-winning sick kids—
the latest inductees into . . .

The Sick Kids Hall of Fame

☆

LEAST HELPFUL PATIENT AWARD

Mark F. Zorro, 10, when examined by his doctor, managed to answer 23 straight questions by saying, "I just don't feel well." When Mark's parents asked the doctor what was wrong with their son, he shrugged his shoulders and said, "I guess he just doesn't feel well!" No one ever did find out what Mark's problem was.

☆

MOST CHICKEN SOUP CONSUMPTION AWARD

Chris P. Chicken, 10, on a November Tuesday, consumed exactly 12½ gallons of chicken soup. Chris said he could have eaten more, but he wants to save some in case he gets sick again.

☆

BEST SICKBED ARRANGEMENT AWARD

Mike Lockisfast, 10, took seven hours and thirty-five minutes to rearrange his pillow 143 times before he got it just the way he wanted it. Once he had settled back, he realized that his blankets weren't arranged properly. By the time Mike got his bed to his liking, he wasn't sick anymore!

☆

BEST PILL SWALLOWER AWARD

Benton Destruction, 13, claims that, unlike most other people, he has no trouble whatsoever swallowing pills. Benton says that to make pill swallowing more challenging, he never uses water and often has a mouthful of crackers at swallowing time. Benton claims that he holds the world's record for once swallowing a pill that was larger than his head! (Benton's friends say that he holds the world's record for telling ridiculous stories!)

☆

QUIETEST COUGH AWARD

Marge Inforerror, 12, who is always most polite and proper, has mastered the polite and proper Quiet Cough. No matter how sick she gets, Marge coughs quietly into her pillow so as not to disturb her parents. As a result, her parents lie awake all night wondering whether she is coughing or not!

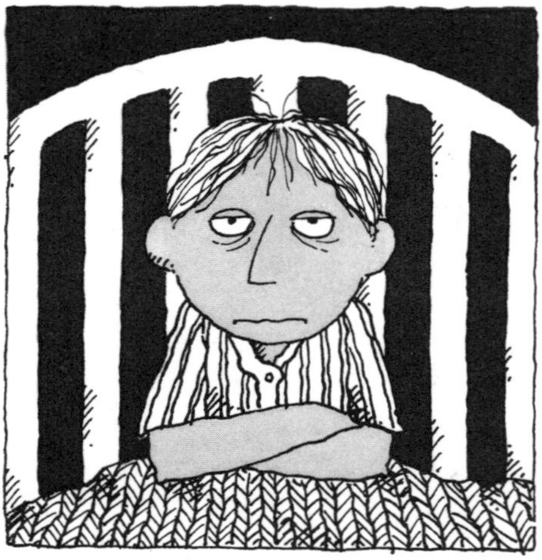

LEAST HELPFUL PATIENT

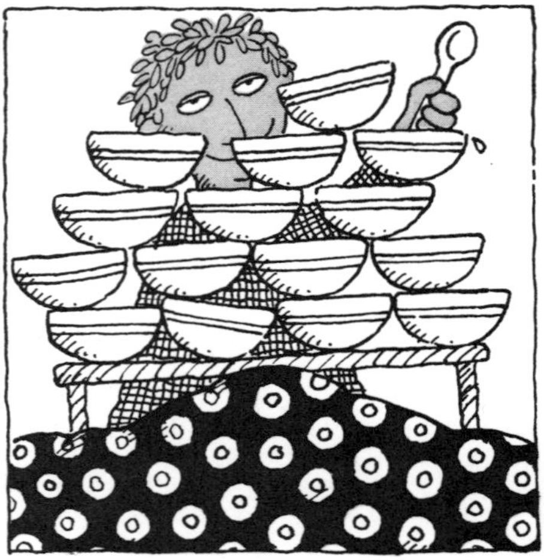

MOST CHICKEN SOUP CONSUMPTION

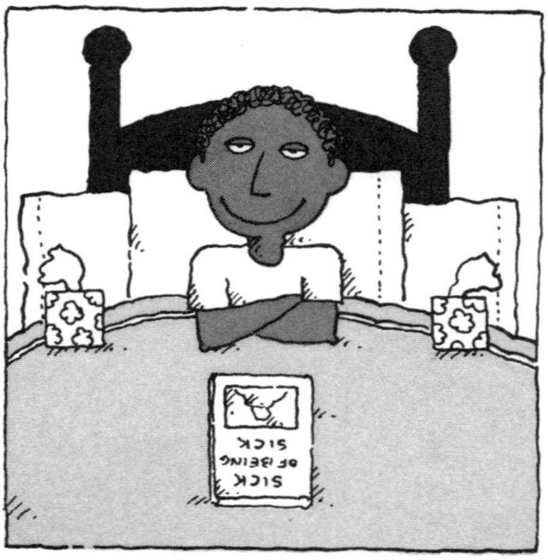

BEST SICKBED ARRANGEMENT

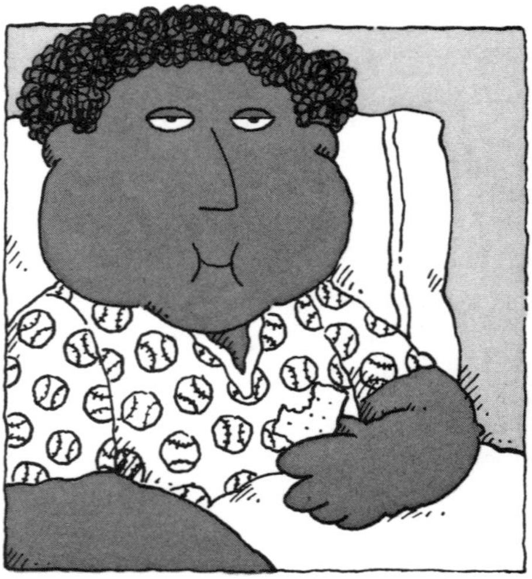

BEST PILL SWALLOWER

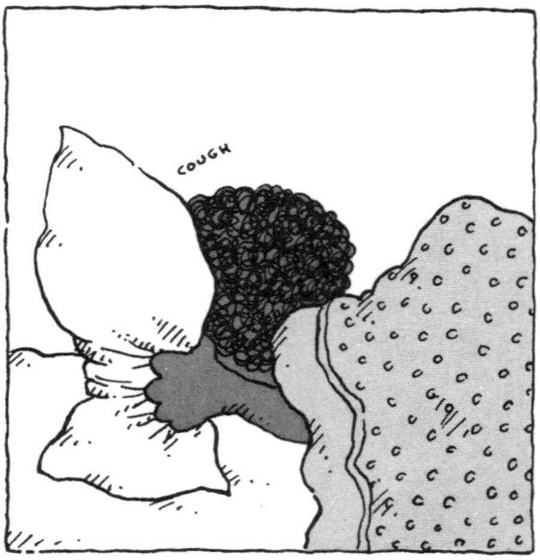

QUIETEST COUGH

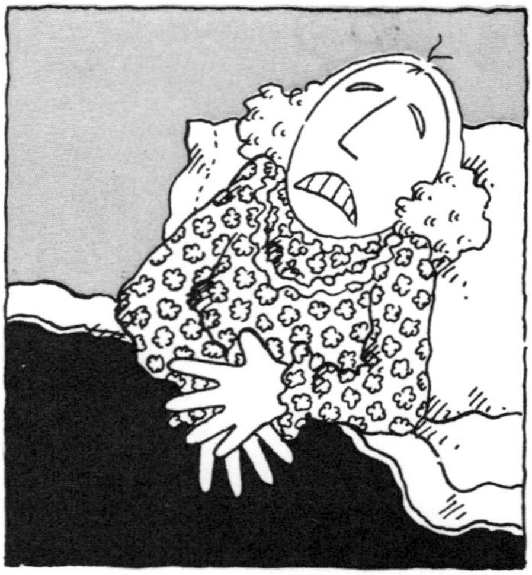

BEST COMPLAINER

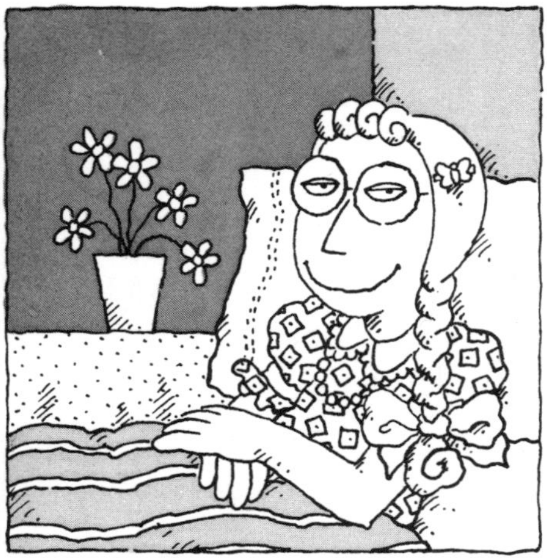

BEST DRESSED

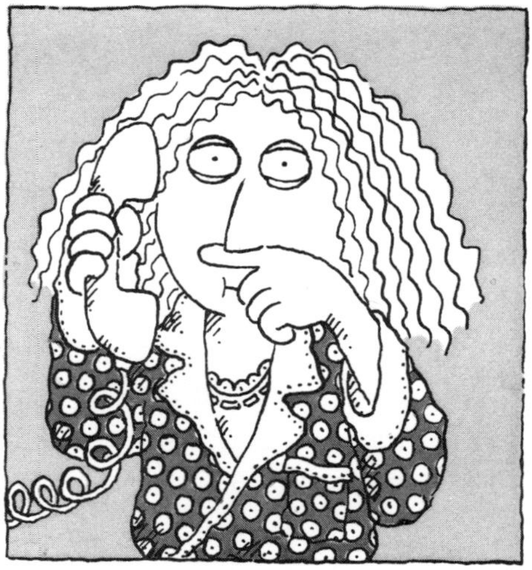

LONG-DISTANCE SNEEZE

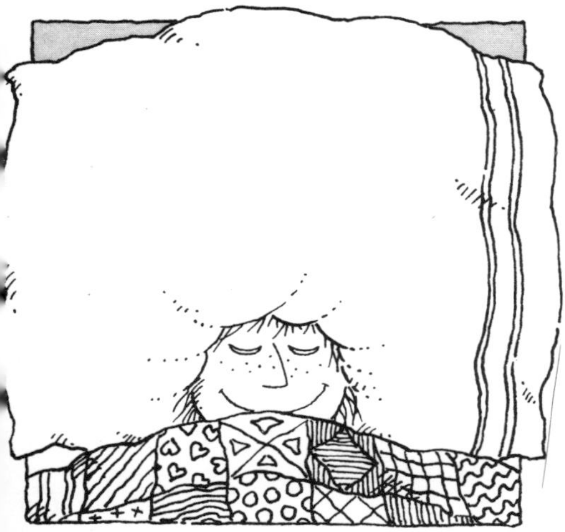

BEST PILLOW FLUFFER-UPPER

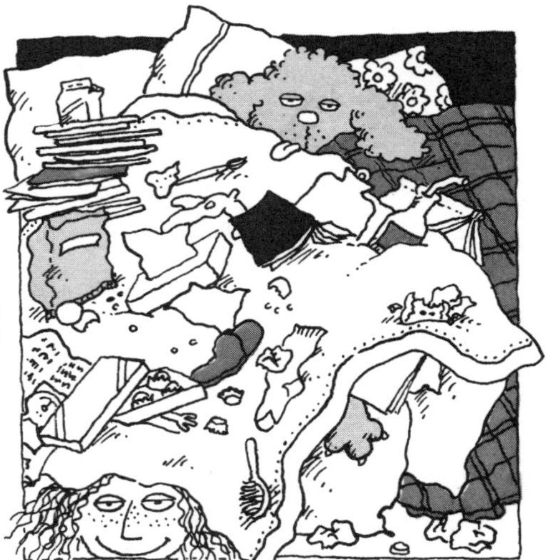

MOST CLUTTERED BED

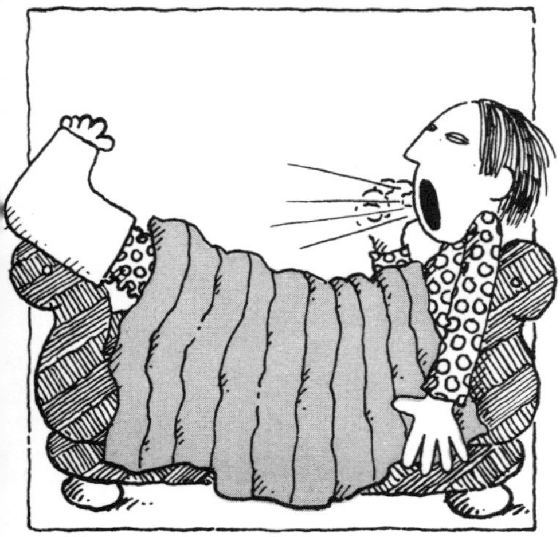

BEST UNNECESSARY COUGH

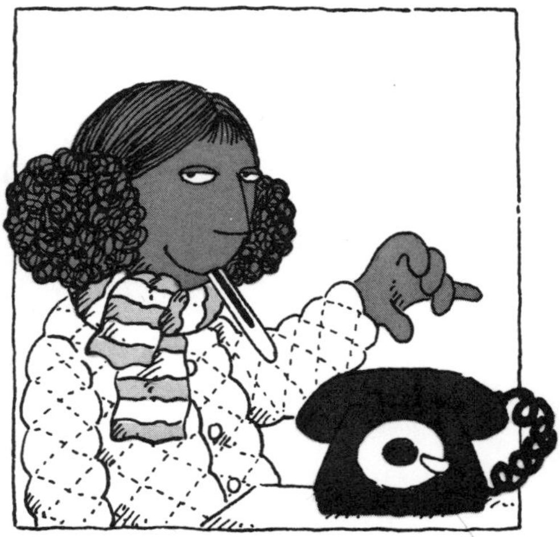

BEST THERMOMETER TALKING

☆

BEST COMPLAINER AWARD

Nina Pinta Santa Maria, 12, broke all records by coming up with 324 different ways to complain about a stomach ache—without once gesturing with her hands! Some day in the future, Nina hopes to write a novel in which every character has a stomach ache.

☆

BEST-DRESSED AWARD

Jan U. Arrymarch, 9, insisted on wearing only her best clothes, even though she was sick in bed. By the time she got well, there was nothing left in her closet, and she was forced to go to school in her pajamas!

☆

LONG-DISTANCE SNEEZE AWARD

April Foole, 11, broke all existing records by sneezing more than 3,000 miles. April lives in New Jersey, and at the time of the sneeze she was on the phone, talking to her grandmother in California! (April says she is practicing so that someday she may make a transatlantic sneeze.)

☆

BEST PILLOW FLUFFER-UPPER AWARD

Art Gum-Eraser III, 12, is known far and wide (mostly wide) as the best pillow fluffer-upper in the nation. When he's sick, Art will not rest until he has fluffed up his pillow at least to the size of a sofa cushion. During a recent illness, Art set a world's record by fluffing up his pillow so big that it didn't fit in his room and his family had to move to a bigger house!

☆

MOST CLUTTERED BED AWARD

Alice N. Wonderland, 12, filled her bed with 324 puzzle books, 783 magazines, 400 games, 6 decks of cards, 120 boxes of tissues, 40 boxes of crackers and cookies, and her Saint Bernard. When her parents came up to see if she needed anything, it took them two days to find her!

☆

BEST UNNECESSARY COUGH AWARD

Bartlett Pear, 11, impressed everyone with an award-winning honking cough that ended in a high-pitched wheeze. Bartlett demonstrated the cough once every ten seconds—despite the fact that he was suffering from a sprained ankle!

☆

BEST THERMOMETER-TALKING AWARD

Dawn Talksomuch, 12, set a new world's record by talking on the phone to a friend for three hours and twelve minutes without ever removing the thermometer from under her tongue. Unfortunately, Dawn's friend couldn't understand a single word she said!

A Get Well Card
for You

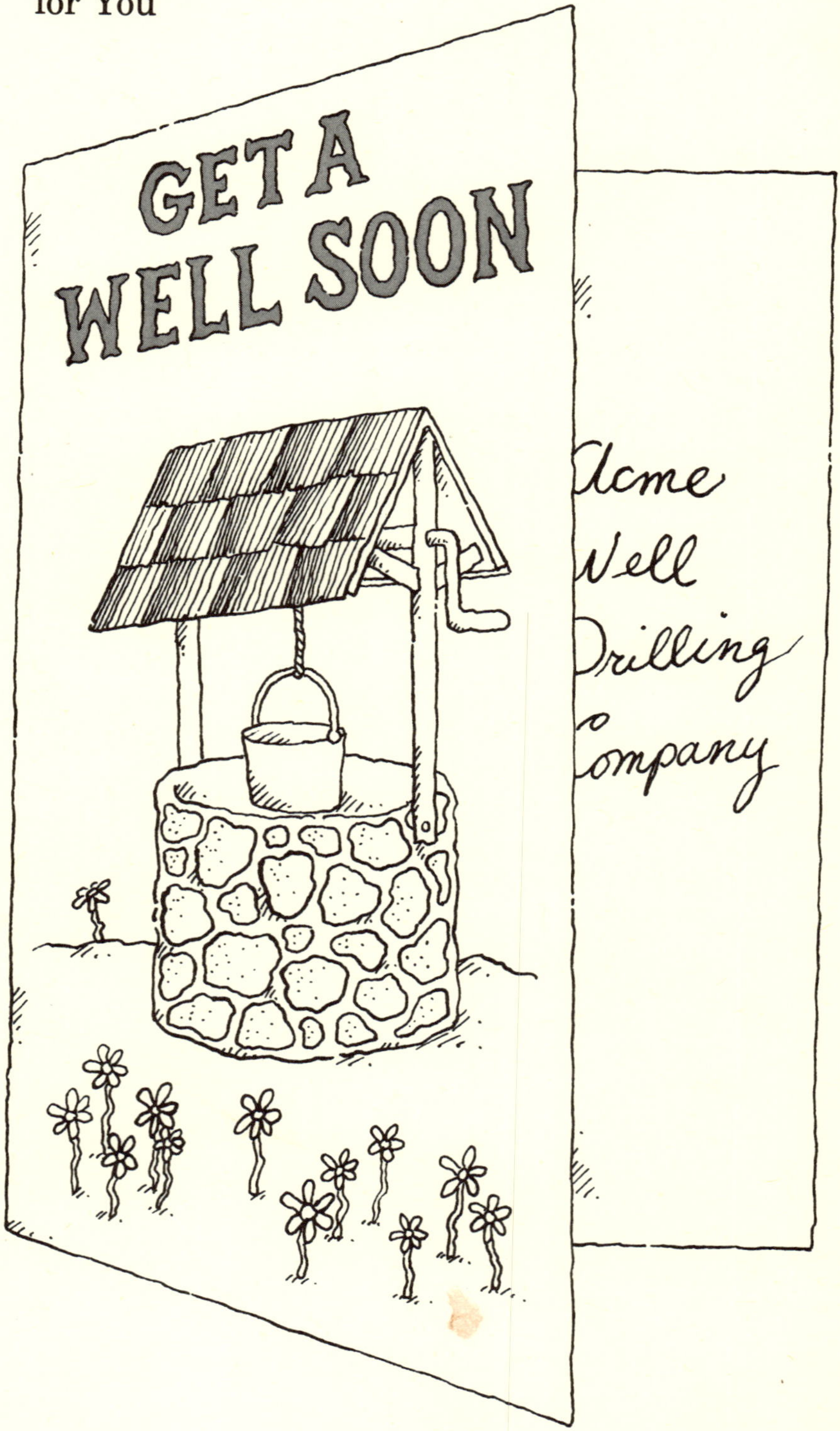

Don't Just Lie There—
Do Something! (#4)

10 Terrible Torturous Tongue Twisters

Tell the truth—couldn't you use a little exercise? Maybe you're not up to your usual 100 sit-ups, but that doesn't mean you have to go completely soft. You can limber up your tongue with these tongue-tying tongue twisters. Once you've got them down pat, you'll be the champ as you challenge all your visitors to the tongue-tangliest tongue-twister tournament of all time!

Go ahead—try these:

- Truly rural, truly rural, truly rural.
- Six slim slick slender saplings.
- Lemon liniment, lemon liniment, lemon liniment.
- This is a zither. This is a zither.
- The swan swam under the swell. Swim, swan, swim.
- Preshrunk shirts, preshrunk shirts, preshrunk shirts.
- The successful thistle sifter sifted his thistles through his sieve and sifter.
- Mister Basket, biscuit mixer. Mister Basket, biscuit mixer.
- Sticky statistics, sticky statistics.
- The sixth sick sheik's sixth sheep's sick.*

* This is supposed to be the hardest tongue twister in the English language.

Other Sick Books You May Enjoy

101 Coughing Games by Ann Gree Hacker

Here are rules for 101 delightful coughing games that can be played by two to four coughers, or by an entire coughing party. Games range from the simple Cough on Mommy to the more challenging Cough Charades.

Raging Fever by Ray Gene Feever

In this less-than-useful guidebook, the author describes the best ways to get a raging fever, how to keep your fever raging, and how to try for record-high fevers despite your body's attempts to get well. The chapter on tossing and turning is excellent, while the chapter on chills is not so hot.

Making the Best of Boils Author Unknown

This perennial sickroom favorite offers a sometimes hilarious, sometimes painful tribute to boils. The anonymous author's advice to "try to go on living despite them" has inspired many a sufferer. Lots of illustrations.

Man With the Million-Dollar Sneeze by Hank R. Cheef

By now, we all know the heartwarming story of how the author turned a single sneeze into a million-dollar fortune. But this retelling of the story in rhyme is utterly charming. Soon to be a major movie disappointment.

First Guide to Doctor Biting by Chu Litely

Doctor biting becomes more popular each year in the United States, and this easy-to-follow guide will have you biting your doctor with ease and skill in no time. Wrist nips, shoulder chomps, back bites—they're all here. Enjoy!

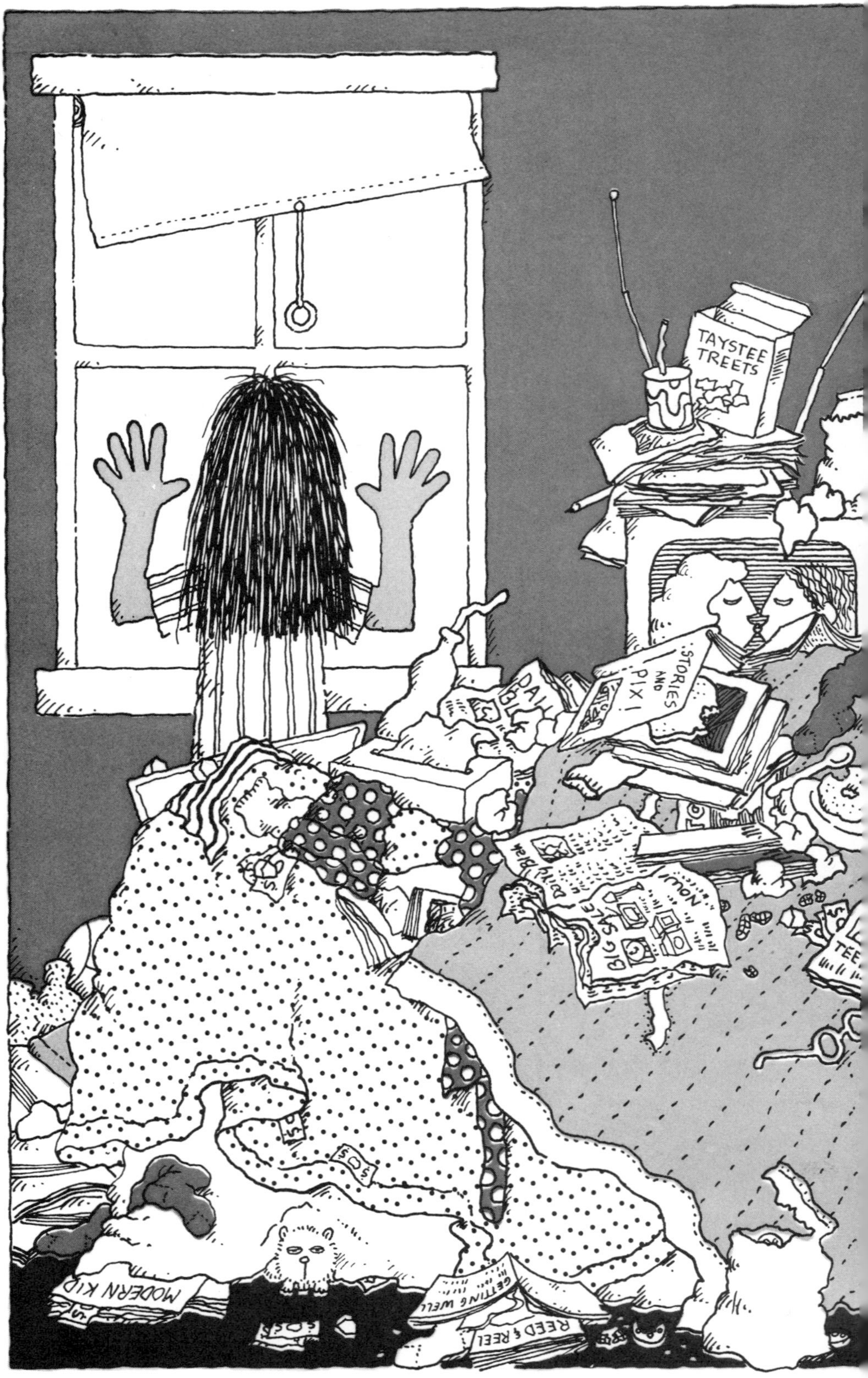
TAYSTEE TREETS
STORIES AND PIX!
BIG SALE NOW!
MODERN KID
GETTING WELL
REED & REEL

Is It Time To Go Back to School? Test Yourself!

1. Count your ears. Do you see two of them? If so, there's something wrong with your eyes. Most people can't see their ears!
2. Stick out your tongue and say *cheese*.
3. Are you beginning to care whether Roger and Marsha will find happiness on "Love of Soap"? Quick—get out of bed if it isn't already too late!
4. Count your hair. If you count more than 648,000 hairs, you must be either very weird or very bored. Get out of bed and find something more constructive to do!
5. Do you have a ringing in your ears? If a man answers, hang up!
6. Close your eyes. Did everything go black? (Be sure to open your eyes before you go on to the next question.)
7. Stand up. Did your pajama bottoms fall to your ankles? If so, you may be suffering from a severe peanut-butter-and-jelly deficiency. Quick—run to the kitchen to remedy this situation!
8. Sneeze three times.
9. Gesundheit. Gesundheit. Gesundheit!

10. Read this joke:

"Doctor, my husband thinks he's a chicken. It's been going on for a month now."

"A month? Why didn't you call me sooner?"

"I would have—but we needed the eggs!"

If you're in such bad shape that you laughed at this tired old joke, you need at least another week in bed!

11. Take a survey of your bed. Can you find more than 82 books and magazines, 7 half-eaten sandwiches, 42 Monopoly pieces, a live gopher, and 12 pairs of purple socks? If so, you have gone over the legal limit. Vacate the premises immediately!

12. Get up, stand on one foot, wave your arms above your head, bend over backwards, and quack like a duck. Now, don't you feel ridiculous? Go on to the next question. We won't tell anyone about this embarrassing incident if you won't!

13. Sit up. Is your pillow still attached to the back of your head? Get out of bed quick before it has to be removed surgically!

14. Did you find this test funny? Yes? Poor thing—you've definitely been in bed too long! Have a nice day in school!

JOVIAL BOB STINE and JANE STINE wrote *The Sick of Being Sick Book* because "sick kids need a good, healthy laugh more than anyone! Most books for kids who are sick in bed try to take the kids' minds off their illness. But we figured you're only sick two or three times a year—why not make the most of it? And we think that concentrating on being sick is bound to make you so sick of being sick that you just have to get better!"

Getting sick may not be a kid's idea of fun, but *The Sick of Being Sick Book* will at least help to make it funny!

Bob and Jane live in New York City.

CAROL NICKLAUS says that illustrating this book gave her a chance "to do work with a bit more sophistication and a touch of the—forgive me—'sick.'"

She first worked with Jovial Bob on Ohio State University's humor magazine, *The Sundial,* where he was editor and she was art editor. Since then, she has illustrated *How To Be Funny* and forty other books, including several she has written herself.

Ms. Nicklaus and her husband live in Danbury, Connecticut.